The BODYBLISS Protocol Journal
Effortlessly Attain and Maintain Your Ideal Weight Forever

Copyright © 2020 Sara Palmer Hussey

The BODYBLISS Protocol Journal is the perfect companion to *The BODYBLISS Protocol*. Having absorbed the teachings in *The BODYBLISS Protocol*, you will now have a new framework for weight management. You now know that when and why you eat is just as important as what you eat. You have redefined your health and lifestyle around the four pillars of successful weight management: timing (keeping eating within a maximum time window of twelve hours and prioritising good sleep), mindset (balancing stress and replacing addictive patterns with healthy modalities), nutrition (learning to nourish the body with the healthiest, most nutrient-rich meals) and metabolism (developing a strong metabolism through exercise and cold exposure).

The BODYBLISS Protocol Journal will pave the way for the healthiest relationship with your body, teaching you to respect it and give it your best care. It nurtures thankfulness for all the wonderful ways in which your body facilitates your experience of life and carries you through this journey. *The BODYBLISS Protocol* experience is not about conforming to a specific body size or shape; it is about cultivating the best health of your unique body, leaving aside restrictive diets and gruelling exercise routines and developing instead an attitude of care and appreciation for your marvellous body. Through application of *The BODYBLISS Protocol*, it is effortless to attain and maintain your optimum weight, which is a healthy weight that feels comfortable, liberating and promotes maximum body confidence.

The BODYBLISS Protocol is the system you have been looking for, the system that will finally make weight management so easy that you no longer have to even think about it and you can just get on with your life. In order for this to be true, we have to engage with the subconscious mind to such an extent that this system becomes an automatic habit. This is achieved by creating habitual behaviour. *The BODYBLISS Protocol Journal* is the habit-forming tool recommended to engage with your subconscious mind and turn this system into second nature for you.

It is believed that any behaviour requires between a few and several weeks of assiduous practice before it can become an ingrained habit. *The BODYBLISS Protocol Journal* gives you the framework to keep tabs on your compliance, track your progress and highlight any issues. Once a week, you will be given the opportunity to review your progress, course correct, if necessary, recalibrate your focus and plot your direction for the week ahead.

Each day you will enter your weight at the top of the page. This is a tracking exercise that confirms your progress, your stability or provides an early warning detection point if you are starting to veer off course. Your weight can fluctuate from day to day, but a steady increase or decrease over the course of a week usually highlights a trend. The journal allows you to look back over the last week to identify the elements that may have contributed to this trend.

The TIMING box firstly asks about your sleep. Did you sleep well? This is a yes or no answer. If the answer is no, you might want to check what elements from the day before may have contributed to not getting a good night's sleep. Did you go to bed later than usual? Did you have dinner later than usual? Were you more stressed than usual? Did you sit up watching television? If you are a woman, could it be that you are premenstrual? How can you ensure that you will sleep better tonight?

The rest of the TIMING box entries refer to times: What time did you have breakfast? What time did you finish dinner? How many hours was your eating window (completion of dinnertime minus breakfast time, eg. 19h (7pm) – 8h (8am) = 11 hours)? What time did you switch off all screens? What time did you go to bed?

The MINDSET box requires more thought. You can use this section to plan your day and record what you achieved. So, for relaxation, list the activities you will engage in to counterbalance any stress in your day. Examples might include yoga, a walk by the sea and meditation. Your list can be the plan and then you can tick off what you actually did. The mindful eating entry is an assessment of whether you ate your meals mindfully without doing some other activity at the same time. Two ticks and a cross would mean you practised mindful eating during two meals, but combined eating with something else on the third meal.

The gratitude list allows space for you to keep note of what you are most grateful for in your life. It can be something different every day or the same, but always take a moment to fully feel your appreciation and thankfulness for every entry on your list.

Self-care and kindness refers to the ways in which you are looking after yourself. If you are someone who takes care of everyone else before you think of yourself, this section forces you to find ways each day to be kind and caring to yourself too. There may be some crossover between this and other sections of the MINDSET box, but try to really use this list to start to identify all the ways in which you can be more caring and kind towards yourself.

The visualisation entry is to check whether you completed a visualisation exercise. Take some time with this; make it a fun, enjoyable experience. The more emotional input you pour into imagining yourself at your best, the more compelled you will be to match this vision for yourself in reality.

The creativity/joy/fun entry is to check whether you are developing your sense of passion and adventure. This section is just for fun. Did you listen to some of your favourite music? Did you sing and dance? Did you knit, doodle, paint, cook, write or draw just for the fun of it with no pressure to be any good? Did you explore some topic just to discover more about it? Did you make a daisy chain? Did you play with your kids? All these activities feed your soul and add to your happiness quota.

The connection/love list ensures that you are in touch with others, people you love and care for. Did you call your parents? Did you send your best friend a message? Did you invite a friend round for dinner? How did you express your love for someone today? Cultivating connection and love is a big reason why we are all here. By prioritising this aspect of our lives and checking in with it every day, we ensure that the busy-ness of life does not obscure what is really important.

The priorities/focus/purpose/service list allows us to define what, if we completed, would give us a sense of achievement and purpose. This can be something relating to work, to a hobby, to your family and friends; whatever is really important for you to do today goes here. Examples might include clearing out the spare room, completing a specific work project, accompanying your daughter to her hockey match, writing a poem or calling someone about a work opportunity. These are all actions that you prioritise that move in the direction of your purpose. Tick off the ones you completed to reinforce a sense of satisfaction and reevaluate those that were not completed; do they require more time? Do you need to add them to the next day? Are they not that important to you? Can you remove them to make room for something of more value to you?

In the NUTRITION box, you record how many times you ate and check or cross whether you included a good source of protein in your meals, whether you ate fruit and vegetables, healthy fat, fibre, whether you drank some diluted apple cider vinegar before at least one meal and whether you remembered to take your supplements. This box purposefully requires a low input from you. It intentionally shifts the focus away from exactly what you ate to whether you sufficiently nourished your body. Your focus is on building a valuable life, not on keeping track of calories.

In the METABOLISM box, you can keep track of whether you are doing everything you can to support a healthy metabolism, cardiovascular health, flexibility and high energy. The first entry is a yes or no response to whether you had any cold exposure; did you give yourself a cold blast under the shower? Did you go for a swim in the sea? The aerobic entry might be a 20-minute walk to work, for example, a vigorous dance session or a jog around the block. For the anaerobic exercise section, seven lines are given to enter which HIIT exercises you completed (a full list of exercises is given below for reference). The flexibility exercise entry might read stretching, a few yoga poses or a full yoga class.

HIIT Exercises

Upper Body
Section 1
1. Plank Jacks (jump legs out to side and back)
2. Plank to Downward Dog
3. Lateral plank walk
4. Plank with shoulder taps
5. Plank to Push up
6. Plank with Arm extensions
7. Straight Plank

Section 2
1. Tricep Dips in crab position or off a chair
2. Bicep curls with weights
3. Push ups
4. Punch Ball on both sides
5. Arm Rotations with weights (arms outstretched)
6. Superman

7. Arm Lifts

Legs and Glutes

Section 3
1. Squats
2. Lunges
3. Reverse Lunges
4. Side lunges
5. 30 Plies with 30 pulses
6. Forward leg lifts
7. Backward Leg lifts

Section 4
1. Jumping Jacks
2. Karate kicks
3. Squat kicks
4. Squat jumps (touch floor and up)
5. Burpee squats
6. Speed Skater
7. Mountain Climber

Section 5
1. Glute bridge
2. Side Leg Lifts
3. Inner Thigh Lifts
4. Donkey kicks
5. Wide-leg glute bridge
6. Side donkey kicks
7. Seated to glute bridge

Abs

Section 6
1. Elbow to knee crunches
2. Russian twist
3. Heel taps
4. Alternating toe touches
5. Side plank dips
6. Plank with knee tucks

7. Dead bug
Section 7
   1. Flutter Kicks
   2. Sit-ups
   3. Extension to Cannonball
   4. V-Ups
   5. Crunches
   6. Reach Crunches
   7. Leg Lifts

Every seventh day in *The BODYBLISS Protocol Journal*, you have a chance to review your progress and study what changes you would like to make for the week ahead. *The BODYBLISS Protocol Journal* allows you to plan in advance, determine your focus for the week, align with your goals and celebrate those goals achieved.

Now that we have the tools for making weight management easy, our health and weight no longer requires our obsessive attention. *The BODYBLISS Protocol* has hopefully freed our attention from the all-consuming obsession of weight-watching and allowed us to rediscover what we really want our lives to be about. *The BODYBLISS Protocol Journal* can really help us keep aligned with that new focus every day while moving towards ever better health and effortless weight management.

The BODYBLISS Protocol Journal offers you 25 weeks to transform your life.

Enjoy the journey!

"The journey of a thousand miles
begins with one step."

Lao Tzu

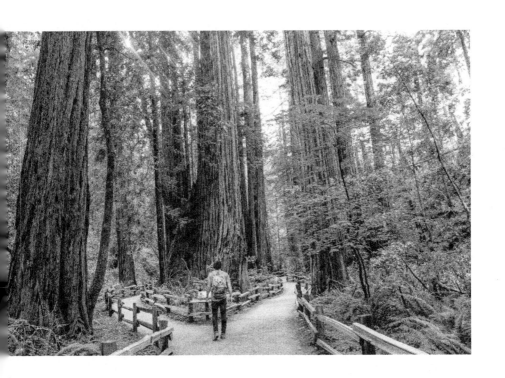

TIMING

A Good Night's Sleep YES/NO

Breakfast............................

Dinner Completed...............

Window...........................

Digital Curfew...................

Bedtime...........................

MINDSET

Relaxation

....

....

Mindful Eating   YES/NO

Gratitude

....

....

....

Self-care & Kindness

....

....

Visualisation   YES/NO

Creativity/Joy/Fun

....

....

Connection/Love

....

....

Priorities/Focus/Purpose

....

....

....

....

Date:................................

Weight:......................

NUTRITION

Number of Meals.............

Protein   YES/NO

Fruit & vegetables   YES/NO

Healthy Fat   YES/NO

Fibre   YES/NO

Apple Cider Vinegar   YES/NO

Supplements   YES/NO

METABOLISM

Cold Exposure   YES/NO

Aerobic Exercise

   ✓ ....

   ✓ ....

Anaerobic Exercise

   ✓ ....

   ✓ ....

   ✓ ....

   ✓ ....

   ✓ ....

   ✓ ....

   ✓ ....

Flexibility Exercise

   ✓ ....

   ✓ ....

TIMING

A Good Night's Sleep YES/NO

Breakfast............................

Dinner Completed..............

Window...........................

Digital Curfew...................

Bedtime...........................

MINDSET

Relaxation
....
....

Mindful Eating   YES/NO

Gratitude
....
....
....

Self-care & Kindness
....
....

Visualisation   YES/NO

Creativity/Joy/Fun
....
....

Connection/Love
....
....

Priorities/Focus/Purpose
....
....
....
....

Date:.................................

Weight:......................

NUTRITION

Number of Meals.............

Protein	YES/NO
Fruit & vegetables	YES/NO
Healthy Fat	YES/NO
Fibre	YES/NO
Apple Cider Vinegar	YES/NO
Supplements	YES/NO

METABOLISM

Cold Exposure   YES/NO

Aerobic Exercise
✓ ....
✓ ....

Anaerobic Exercise
✓ ....
✓ ....
✓ ....
✓ ....
✓ ....
✓ ....
✓ ....

Flexibility Exercise
✓ ....
✓ ....

TIMING

A Good Night's Sleep YES/NO

Breakfast..........................

Dinner Completed...............

Window...........................

Digital Curfew...................

Bedtime...........................

MINDSET

Relaxation
....
....

Mindful Eating   YES/NO

Gratitude
....
....
....

Self-care & Kindness
....
....

Visualisation   YES/NO

Creativity/Joy/Fun
....
....

Connection/Love
....
....

Priorities/Focus/Purpose
....
....
....
....

Date:..............................

Weight:......................

NUTRITION

Number of Meals............

Protein   YES/NO

Fruit & vegetables   YES/NO

Healthy Fat   YES/NO

Fibre   YES/NO

Apple Cider Vinegar   YES/NO

Supplements   YES/NO

METABOLISM

Cold Exposure   YES/NO

Aerobic Exercise
    ✓   ....
    ✓   ....

Anaerobic Exercise
    ✓   ....
    ✓   ....
    ✓   ....
    ✓   ....
    ✓   ....
    ✓   ....
    ✓   ....

Flexibility Exercise
    ✓   ....
    ✓   ....

TIMING

A Good Night's Sleep YES/NO

Breakfast...........................

Dinner Completed...............

Window...........................

Digital Curfew...................

Bedtime...........................

MINDSET

Relaxation

....
....

Mindful Eating   YES/NO

Gratitude

....
....
....

Self-care & Kindness

....
....

Visualisation   YES/NO

Creativity/Joy/Fun

....
....

Connection/Love

....
....

Priorities/Focus/Purpose

....
....
....
....

Date:................................

Weight:.......................

NUTRITION

Number of Meals............

Protein	YES/NO
Fruit & vegetables	YES/NO
Healthy Fat	YES/NO
Fibre	YES/NO
Apple Cider Vinegar	YES/NO
Supplements	YES/NO

METABOLISM

Cold Exposure   YES/NO

Aerobic Exercise

✓   ....
✓   ....

Anaerobic Exercise

✓   ....
✓   ....
✓   ....
✓   ....
✓   ....
✓   ....
✓   ....

Flexibility Exercise

✓   ....
✓   ....

TIMING

A Good Night's Sleep YES/NO

Breakfast............................

Dinner Completed...............

Window..........................

Digital Curfew...................

Bedtime...........................

MINDSET

Relaxation

....

....

Mindful Eating   YES/NO

Gratitude

....

....

....

Self-care & Kindness

....

....

Visualisation   YES/NO

Creativity/Joy/Fun

....

....

Connection/Love

....

....

Priorities/Focus/Purpose

....

....

....

....

Date:.................................

Weight:........................

NUTRITION

Number of Meals............

Protein	YES/NO
Fruit & vegetables	YES/NO
Healthy Fat	YES/NO
Fibre	YES/NO
Apple Cider Vinegar	YES/NO
Supplements	YES/NO

METABOLISM

Cold Exposure   YES/NO

Aerobic Exercise

✓   ....
✓   ....

Anaerobic Exercise

✓   ....
✓   ....
✓   ....
✓   ....
✓   ....
✓   ....
✓   ....

Flexibility Exercise

✓   ....
✓   ....

TIMING

A Good Night's Sleep YES/NO

Breakfast.............................

Dinner Completed...............

Window............................

Digital Curfew...................

Bedtime............................

MINDSET

Relaxation

....

....

Mindful Eating   YES/NO

Gratitude

....

....

....

Self-care & Kindness

....

....

Visualisation   YES/NO

Creativity/Joy/Fun

....

....

Connection/Love

....

....

Priorities/Focus/Purpose

....

....

....

....

Date:................................

Weight:........................

NUTRITION

Number of Meals............

Protein	YES/NO
Fruit & vegetables	YES/NO
Healthy Fat	YES/NO
Fibre	YES/NO
Apple Cider Vinegar	YES/NO
Supplements	YES/NO

METABOLISM

Cold Exposure   YES/NO

Aerobic Exercise

✓   ....

✓   ....

Anaerobic Exercise

✓   ....

✓   ....

✓   ....

✓   ....

✓   ....

✓   ....

✓   ....

Flexibility Exercise

✓   ....

✓   ....

TIMING

A Good Night's Sleep YES/NO

Breakfast...........................

Dinner Completed...............

Window...........................

Digital Curfew...................

Bedtime...........................

MINDSET

Relaxation
....
....

Mindful Eating   YES/NO

Gratitude
....
....
....

Self-care & Kindness
....
....

Visualisation   YES/NO

Creativity/Joy/Fun
....
....

Connection/Love
....
....

Priorities/Focus/Purpose
....
....
....
....

Date:..............................

Weight:.......................

NUTRITION

Number of Meals............

Protein   YES/NO

Fruit & vegetables   YES/NO

Healthy Fat   YES/NO

Fibre   YES/NO

Apple Cider Vinegar   YES/NO

Supplements   YES/NO

METABOLISM

Cold Exposure   YES/NO

Aerobic Exercise
✓   ....
✓   ....

Anaerobic Exercise
✓   ....
✓   ....
✓   ....
✓   ....
✓   ....
✓   ....
✓   ....

Flexibility Exercise
✓   ....
✓   ....

WEEKLY REVIEW

Weight:	Weight:
Review...............................	Focus...............................

TIMING:	TIMING:
Review................................	Focus................................
....	....
....	....
....	....
....	....

MINDSET:	MINDSET:
Review................................	Focus................................
....	....
....	....
....	....
....	....
....	....
....	....

NUTRITION:	NUTRITION:
Review	Focus................................
....	....
....	....
....	....
....	....
....	....

METABOLISM:	METABOLISM:
Review................................	Focus................................
....	....
....	....
....	....
....	....

"When you arise in the morning, think of what a precious privilege it is to be alive - to breathe, to think, to enjoy, to love."

Marcus Aurelius

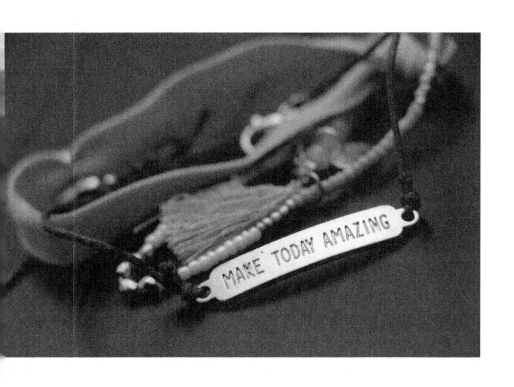

TIMING

A Good Night's Sleep YES/NO

Breakfast...........................

Dinner Completed...............

Window...........................

Digital Curfew....................

Bedtime...........................

MINDSET

Relaxation

....

....

Mindful Eating   YES/NO

Gratitude

....

....

....

Self-care & Kindness

....

....

Visualisation   YES/NO

Creativity/Joy/Fun

....

....

Connection/Love

....

....

Priorities/Focus/Purpose

....

....

....

....

Date:................................

Weight:......................

NUTRITION

Number of Meals............

Protein	YES/NO
Fruit & vegetables	YES/NO
Healthy Fat	YES/NO
Fibre	YES/NO
Apple Cider Vinegar	YES/NO
Supplements	YES/NO

METABOLISM

Cold Exposure   YES/NO

Aerobic Exercise

✓   ....

✓   ....

Anaerobic Exercise

✓   ....

✓   ....

✓   ....

✓   ....

✓   ....

✓   ....

✓   ....

Flexibility Exercise

✓   ....

✓   ....

TIMING

A Good Night's Sleep YES/NO

Breakfast...........................

Dinner Completed..............

Window...........................

Digital Curfew...................

Bedtime...........................

MINDSET

Relaxation

....
....

Mindful Eating   YES/NO

Gratitude

....
....
....

Self-care & Kindness

....
....

Visualisation   YES/NO

Creativity/Joy/Fun

....
....

Connection/Love

....
....

Priorities/Focus/Purpose

....
....
....
....

Date:...............................

Weight:.......................

NUTRITION

Number of Meals............

Protein	YES/NO
Fruit & vegetables	YES/NO
Healthy Fat	YES/NO
Fibre	YES/NO
Apple Cider Vinegar	YES/NO
Supplements	YES/NO

METABOLISM

Cold Exposure   YES/NO

Aerobic Exercise

✓   ....
✓   ....

Anaerobic Exercise

✓   ....
✓   ....
✓   ....
✓   ....
✓   ....
✓   ....
✓   ....

Flexibility Exercise

✓   ....
✓   ....

TIMING

A Good Night's Sleep YES/NO

Breakfast...........................

Dinner Completed...............

Window...........................

Digital Curfew...................

Bedtime...........................

MINDSET

Relaxation
....
....

Mindful Eating   YES/NO

Gratitude
....
....
....

Self-care & Kindness
....
....

Visualisation   YES/NO

Creativity/Joy/Fun
....
....

Connection/Love
....
....

Priorities/Focus/Purpose
....
....
....
....

Date:................................

Weight:......................

NUTRITION

Number of Meals.............

Protein	YES/NO
Fruit & vegetables	YES/NO
Healthy Fat	YES/NO
Fibre	YES/NO
Apple Cider Vinegar	YES/NO
Supplements	YES/NO

METABOLISM

Cold Exposure   YES/NO

Aerobic Exercise
   ✓   ....
   ✓   ....

Anaerobic Exercise
   ✓   ....
   ✓   ....
   ✓   ....
   ✓   ....
   ✓   ....
   ✓   ....
   ✓   ....

Flexibility Exercise
   ✓   ....
   ✓   ....

TIMING

A Good Night's Sleep YES/NO

Breakfast...........................

Dinner Completed..............

Window..........................

Digital Curfew...................

Bedtime..........................

MINDSET

Relaxation

....

....

Mindful Eating   YES/NO

Gratitude

....

....

....

Self-care & Kindness

....

....

Visualisation   YES/NO

Creativity/Joy/Fun

....

....

Connection/Love

....

....

Priorities/Focus/Purpose

....

....

....

....

Date:...............................

Weight:.......................

NUTRITION

Number of Meals............

Protein   YES/NO

Fruit & vegetables   YES/NO

Healthy Fat   YES/NO

Fibre   YES/NO

Apple Cider Vinegar   YES/NO

Supplements   YES/NO

METABOLISM

Cold Exposure   YES/NO

Aerobic Exercise

   ✓   ....

   ✓   ....

Anaerobic Exercise

   ✓   ....

   ✓   ....

   ✓   ....

   ✓   ....

   ✓   ....

   ✓   ....

   ✓   ....

Flexibility Exercise

   ✓   ....

   ✓   ....

TIMING

A Good Night's Sleep YES/NO

Breakfast...........................

Dinner Completed...............

Window...........................

Digital Curfew...................

Bedtime...........................

MINDSET

Relaxation
....
....

Mindful Eating   YES/NO

Gratitude
....
....
....

Self-care & Kindness
....
....

Visualisation   YES/NO

Creativity/Joy/Fun
....
....

Connection/Love
....
....

Priorities/Focus/Purpose
....
....
....
....

Date:..............................

Weight:......................

NUTRITION

Number of Meals............

Protein   YES/NO

Fruit & vegetables   YES/NO

Healthy Fat   YES/NO

Fibre   YES/NO

Apple Cider Vinegar   YES/NO

Supplements   YES/NO

METABOLISM

Cold Exposure   YES/NO

Aerobic Exercise

✓   ....
✓   ....

Anaerobic Exercise

✓   ....
✓   ....
✓   ....
✓   ....
✓   ....
✓   ....
✓   ....

Flexibility Exercise

✓   ....
✓   ....

TIMING

A Good Night's Sleep YES/NO

Breakfast...........................

Dinner Completed...............

Window...........................

Digital Curfew...................

Bedtime............................

Date:...............................

Weight:.......................

NUTRITION

Number of Meals............

Protein	YES/NO
Fruit & vegetables	YES/NO
Healthy Fat	YES/NO
Fibre	YES/NO
Apple Cider Vinegar	YES/NO
Supplements	YES/NO

MINDSET

Relaxation
....
....

Mindful Eating   YES/NO

Gratitude
....
....
....

Self-care & Kindness
....
....

Visualisation   YES/NO

Creativity/Joy/Fun
....
....

Connection/Love
....
....

Priorities/Focus/Purpose
....
....
....
....

METABOLISM

Cold Exposure   YES/NO

Aerobic Exercise
  ✓   ....
  ✓   ....

Anaerobic Exercise
  ✓   ....
  ✓   ....
  ✓   ....
  ✓   ....
  ✓   ....
  ✓   ....
  ✓   ....

Flexibility Exercise
  ✓   ....
  ✓   ....

TIMING

A Good Night's Sleep YES/NO

Breakfast...........................

Dinner Completed...............

Window...........................

Digital Curfew...................

Bedtime...........................

MINDSET

Relaxation

....

....

Mindful Eating   YES/NO

Gratitude

....

....

....

Self-care & Kindness

....

....

Visualisation   YES/NO

Creativity/Joy/Fun

....

....

Connection/Love

....

....

Priorities/Focus/Purpose

....

....

....

....

Date:...............................

Weight:.......................

NUTRITION

Number of Meals............

Protein	YES/NO
Fruit & vegetables	YES/NO
Healthy Fat	YES/NO
Fibre	YES/NO
Apple Cider Vinegar	YES/NO
Supplements	YES/NO

METABOLISM

Cold Exposure   YES/NO

Aerobic Exercise

✓ ....

✓ ....

Anaerobic Exercise

✓ ....

✓ ....

✓ ....

✓ ....

✓ ....

✓ ....

✓ ....

Flexibility Exercise

✓ ....

✓ ....

WEEKLY REVIEW

Weight:

Review.................................

Weight:

Focus.................................

TIMING:

Review..............................
....
....
....
....

TIMING:

Focus..............................
....
....
....
....

MINDSET:

Review..............................
....
....
....
....
....
....

MINDSET:

Focus..............................
....
....
....
....
....
....

NUTRITION:

Review ....
....
....
....
....
....

NUTRITION:

Focus..............................
....
....
....
....
....

METABOLISM:

Review..............................
....
....
....
....

METABOLISM:

Focus..............................
....
....
....
....

"It does not matter how slowly you go as long as you do not stop."

Confucius

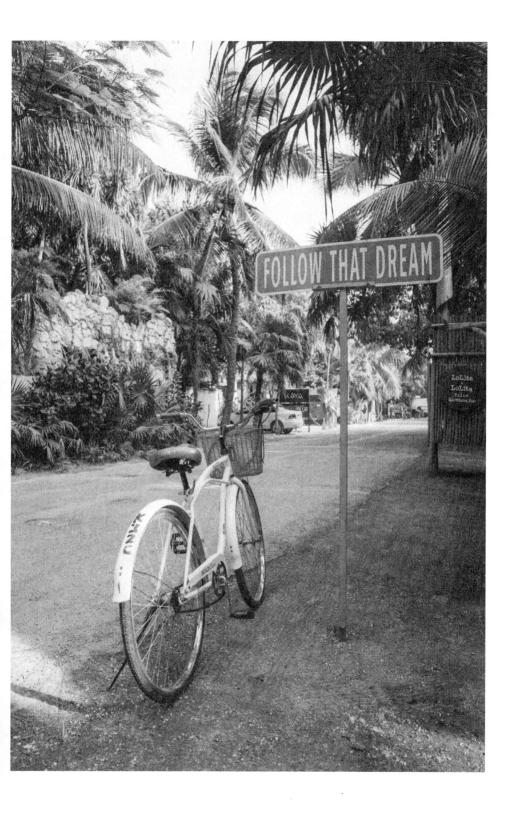

TIMING

A Good Night's Sleep YES/NO

Breakfast...........................

Dinner Completed...............

Window............................

Digital Curfew...................

Bedtime............................

MINDSET

Relaxation

....

....

Mindful Eating   YES/NO

Gratitude

....

....

....

Self-care & Kindness

....

....

Visualisation   YES/NO

Creativity/Joy/Fun

....

....

Connection/Love

....

....

Priorities/Focus/Purpose

....

....

....

....

Date:..................................

Weight:.......................

NUTRITION

Number of Meals............

Protein	YES/NO
Fruit & vegetables	YES/NO
Healthy Fat	YES/NO
Fibre	YES/NO
Apple Cider Vinegar	YES/NO
Supplements	YES/NO

METABOLISM

Cold Exposure   YES/NO

Aerobic Exercise

✓ ....
✓ ....

Anaerobic Exercise

✓ ....
✓ ....
✓ ....
✓ ....
✓ ....
✓ ....
✓ ....

Flexibility Exercise

✓ ....
✓ ....

TIMING

A Good Night's Sleep YES/NO

Breakfast...........................

Dinner Completed...............

Window...........................

Digital Curfew...................

Bedtime...........................

MINDSET

Relaxation
....
....

Mindful Eating   YES/NO

Gratitude
....
....
....

Self-care & Kindness
....
....

Visualisation   YES/NO

Creativity/Joy/Fun
....
....

Connection/Love
....
....

Priorities/Focus/Purpose
....
....
....
....

Date:.................................

Weight:.......................

NUTRITION

Number of Meals............

Protein	YES/NO
Fruit & vegetables	YES/NO
Healthy Fat	YES/NO
Fibre	YES/NO
Apple Cider Vinegar	YES/NO
Supplements	YES/NO

METABOLISM

Cold Exposure   YES/NO

Aerobic Exercise
  ✓ ....
  ✓ ....

Anaerobic Exercise
  ✓ ....
  ✓ ....
  ✓ ....
  ✓ ....
  ✓ ....
  ✓ ....
  ✓ ....

Flexibility Exercise
  ✓ ....
  ✓ ....

TIMING

A Good Night's Sleep YES/NO

Breakfast...........................

Dinner Completed...............

Window...........................

Digital Curfew...................

Bedtime...........................

MINDSET

Relaxation

....
....

Mindful Eating   YES/NO

Gratitude

....
....
....

Self-care & Kindness

....
....

Visualisation   YES/NO

Creativity/Joy/Fun

....
....

Connection/Love

....
....

Priorities/Focus/Purpose

....
....
....
....

Date:...............................

Weight:.......................

NUTRITION

Number of Meals............

Protein	YES/NO
Fruit & vegetables	YES/NO
Healthy Fat	YES/NO
Fibre	YES/NO
Apple Cider Vinegar	YES/NO
Supplements	YES/NO

METABOLISM

Cold Exposure   YES/NO

Aerobic Exercise

✓ ....
✓ ....

Anaerobic Exercise

✓ ....
✓ ....
✓ ....
✓ ....
✓ ....
✓ ....
✓ ....

Flexibility Exercise

✓ ....
✓ ....

TIMING

A Good Night's Sleep YES/NO

Breakfast...........................

Dinner Completed..............

Window...........................

Digital Curfew..................

Bedtime...........................

MINDSET

Relaxation
....
....

Mindful Eating   YES/NO

Gratitude
....
....
....

Self-care & Kindness
....
....

Visualisation   YES/NO

Creativity/Joy/Fun
....
....

Connection/Love
....
....

Priorities/Focus/Purpose
....
....
....
....

Date:...............................

Weight:........................

NUTRITION

Number of Meals............

Protein	YES/NO
Fruit & vegetables	YES/NO
Healthy Fat	YES/NO
Fibre	YES/NO
Apple Cider Vinegar	YES/NO
Supplements	YES/NO

METABOLISM

Cold Exposure   YES/NO

Aerobic Exercise
   ✓ ....
   ✓ ....

Anaerobic Exercise
   ✓ ....
   ✓ ....
   ✓ ....
   ✓ ....
   ✓ ....
   ✓ ....
   ✓ ....

Flexibility Exercise
   ✓ ....
   ✓ ....

TIMING

A Good Night's Sleep YES/NO

Breakfast............................

Dinner Completed...............

Window...........................

Digital Curfew....................

Bedtime...........................

MINDSET

Relaxation

....

....

Mindful Eating   YES/NO

Gratitude

....

....

....

Self-care & Kindness

....

....

Visualisation   YES/NO

Creativity/Joy/Fun

....

....

Connection/Love

....

....

Priorities/Focus/Purpose

....

....

....

....

Date:..............................

Weight:.......................

NUTRITION

Number of Meals.............

Protein   YES/NO

Fruit & vegetables   YES/NO

Healthy Fat   YES/NO

Fibre   YES/NO

Apple Cider Vinegar   YES/NO

Supplements   YES/NO

METABOLISM

Cold Exposure   YES/NO

Aerobic Exercise

   ✓   ....
   ✓   ....

Anaerobic Exercise

   ✓   ....
   ✓   ....
   ✓   ....
   ✓   ....
   ✓   ....
   ✓   ....
   ✓   ....

Flexibility Exercise

   ✓   ....
   ✓   ....

TIMING

A Good Night's Sleep YES/NO

Breakfast..........................

Dinner Completed..............

Window..........................

Digital Curfew..................

Bedtime..........................

MINDSET

Relaxation

....

....

Mindful Eating   YES/NO

Gratitude

....

....

....

Self-care & Kindness

....

....

Visualisation   YES/NO

Creativity/Joy/Fun

....

....

Connection/Love

....

....

Priorities/Focus/Purpose

....

....

....

....

Date:................................

Weight:.......................

NUTRITION

Number of Meals............

Protein   YES/NO

Fruit & vegetables   YES/NO

Healthy Fat   YES/NO

Fibre   YES/NO

Apple Cider Vinegar   YES/NO

Supplements   YES/NO

METABOLISM

Cold Exposure   YES/NO

Aerobic Exercise

✓ ....

✓ ....

Anaerobic Exercise

✓ ....

✓ ....

✓ ....

✓ ....

✓ ....

✓ ....

✓ ....

Flexibility Exercise

✓ ....

✓ ....

TIMING

A Good Night's Sleep YES/NO

Breakfast...........................

Dinner Completed...............

Window............................

Digital Curfew...................

Bedtime............................

MINDSET

Relaxation

....
....

Mindful Eating   YES/NO

Gratitude

....
....
....

Self-care & Kindness

....
....

Visualisation   YES/NO

Creativity/Joy/Fun

....
....

Connection/Love

....
....

Priorities/Focus/Purpose

....
....
....
....

Date:...............................

Weight:.......................

NUTRITION

Number of Meals............

Protein   YES/NO

Fruit & vegetables   YES/NO

Healthy Fat   YES/NO

Fibre   YES/NO

Apple Cider Vinegar   YES/NO

Supplements   YES/NO

METABOLISM

Cold Exposure   YES/NO

Aerobic Exercise

   ✓   ....
   ✓   ....

Anaerobic Exercise

   ✓   ....
   ✓   ....
   ✓   ....
   ✓   ....
   ✓   ....
   ✓   ....
   ✓   ....

Flexibility Exercise

   ✓   ....
   ✓   ....

WEEKLY REVIEW

Weight:	Weight:
Review............................	Focus............................

TIMING:	TIMING:
Review..........................	Focus.............................
....	....
....	....
....	....
....	....

MINDSET:	MINDSET:
Review............................	Focus.............................
....	....
....	....
....	....
....	....
....	....
....	....

NUTRITION:	NUTRITION:
Review	Focus.............................
....	....
....	....
....	....
....	....
....	....

METABOLISM:	METABOLISM:
Review............................	Focus.............................
....	....
....	....
....	....
....	....

"You have brains in your head. You have feet in your shoes. You can steer yourself in any direction you choose. You're on your own, and you know what you know. And you are the guy who'll decide where to go."

Dr. Seuss

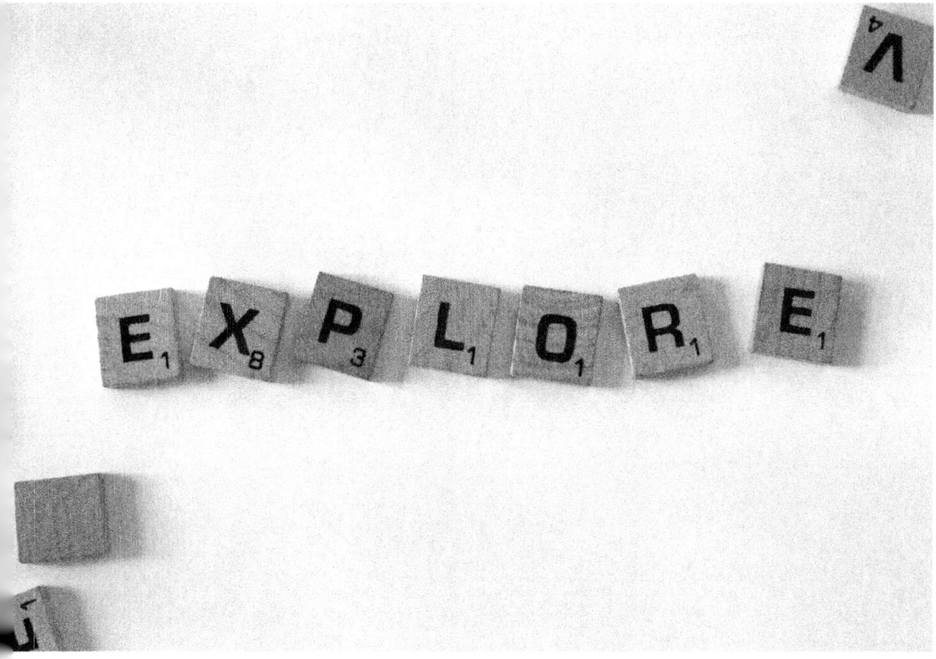
EXPLORE

TIMING

A Good Night's Sleep YES/NO

Breakfast...........................

Dinner Completed...............

Window............................

Digital Curfew....................

Bedtime............................

MINDSET

Relaxation

....

....

Mindful Eating   YES/NO

Gratitude

....

....

....

Self-care & Kindness

....

....

Visualisation   YES/NO

Creativity/Joy/Fun

....

....

Connection/Love

....

....

Priorities/Focus/Purpose

....

....

....

....

Date:...............................

Weight:.......................

NUTRITION

Number of Meals............

Protein   YES/NO

Fruit & vegetables   YES/NO

Healthy Fat   YES/NO

Fibre   YES/NO

Apple Cider Vinegar   YES/NO

Supplements   YES/NO

METABOLISM

Cold Exposure   YES/NO

Aerobic Exercise

   ✓   ....

   ✓   ....

Anaerobic Exercise

   ✓   ....

   ✓   ....

   ✓   ....

   ✓   ....

   ✓   ....

   ✓   ....

   ✓   ....

Flexibility Exercise

   ✓   ....

   ✓   ....

TIMING

A Good Night's Sleep YES/NO

Breakfast...........................

Dinner Completed...............

Window...........................

Digital Curfew...................

Bedtime...........................

MINDSET

Relaxation

....

....

Mindful Eating   YES/NO

Gratitude

....

....

....

Self-care & Kindness

....

....

Visualisation   YES/NO

Creativity/Joy/Fun

....

....

Connection/Love

....

....

Priorities/Focus/Purpose

....

....

....

....

Date:.................................

Weight:.......................

NUTRITION

Number of Meals............

Protein	YES/NO
Fruit & vegetables	YES/NO
Healthy Fat	YES/NO
Fibre	YES/NO
Apple Cider Vinegar	YES/NO
Supplements	YES/NO

METABOLISM

Cold Exposure   YES/NO

Aerobic Exercise

✓   ....
✓   ....

Anaerobic Exercise

✓   ....
✓   ....
✓   ....
✓   ....
✓   ....
✓   ....
✓   ....

Flexibility Exercise

✓   ....
✓   ....

TIMING

A Good Night's Sleep YES/NO

Breakfast............................

Dinner Completed...............

Window...........................

Digital Curfew...................

Bedtime...........................

MINDSET

Relaxation
....
....

Mindful Eating   YES/NO

Gratitude
....
....
....

Self-care & Kindness
....
....

Visualisation   YES/NO

Creativity/Joy/Fun
....
....

Connection/Love
....
....

Priorities/Focus/Purpose
....
....
....
....

Date:...............................

Weight:.......................

NUTRITION

Number of Meals............

Protein   YES/NO

Fruit & vegetables   YES/NO

Healthy Fat   YES/NO

Fibre   YES/NO

Apple Cider Vinegar   YES/NO

Supplements   YES/NO

METABOLISM

Cold Exposure   YES/NO

Aerobic Exercise

   ✓ ....
   ✓ ....

Anaerobic Exercise

   ✓ ....
   ✓ ....
   ✓ ....
   ✓ ....
   ✓ ....
   ✓ ....
   ✓ ....

Flexibility Exercise

   ✓ ....
   ✓ ....

TIMING

A Good Night's Sleep YES/NO

Breakfast...........................

Dinner Completed...............

Window...........................

Digital Curfew...................

Bedtime...........................

MINDSET

Relaxation

....

....

Mindful Eating   YES/NO

Gratitude

....

....

....

Self-care & Kindness

....

....

Visualisation   YES/NO

Creativity/Joy/Fun

....

....

Connection/Love

....

....

Priorities/Focus/Purpose

....

....

....

....

Date:..................................

Weight:.......................

NUTRITION

Number of Meals............

Protein	YES/NO
Fruit & vegetables	YES/NO
Healthy Fat	YES/NO
Fibre	YES/NO
Apple Cider Vinegar	YES/NO
Supplements	YES/NO

METABOLISM

Cold Exposure   YES/NO

Aerobic Exercise

✓   ....

✓   ....

Anaerobic Exercise

✓   ....

✓   ....

✓   ....

✓   ....

✓   ....

✓   ....

✓   ....

Flexibility Exercise

✓   ....

✓   ....

TIMING

A Good Night's Sleep YES/NO

Breakfast...........................

Dinner Completed...............

Window...........................

Digital Curfew...................

Bedtime...........................

MINDSET

Relaxation
....
....

Mindful Eating   YES/NO

Gratitude
....
....
....

Self-care & Kindness
....
....

Visualisation   YES/NO

Creativity/Joy/Fun
....
....

Connection/Love
....
....

Priorities/Focus/Purpose
....
....
....
....

Date:...............................

Weight:......................

NUTRITION

Number of Meals............

Protein	YES/NO
Fruit & vegetables	YES/NO
Healthy Fat	YES/NO
Fibre	YES/NO
Apple Cider Vinegar	YES/NO
Supplements	YES/NO

METABOLISM

Cold Exposure   YES/NO

Aerobic Exercise
- ✓ ....
- ✓ ....

Anaerobic Exercise
- ✓ ....
- ✓ ....
- ✓ ....
- ✓ ....
- ✓ ....
- ✓ ....
- ✓ ....

Flexibility Exercise
- ✓ ....
- ✓ ....

TIMING

A Good Night's Sleep YES/NO

Breakfast...........................

Dinner Completed...............

Window...........................

Digital Curfew...................

Bedtime...........................

MINDSET

Relaxation
....
....

Mindful Eating   YES/NO

Gratitude
....
....
....

Self-care & Kindness
....
....

Visualisation   YES/NO

Creativity/Joy/Fun
....
....

Connection/Love
....
....

Priorities/Focus/Purpose
....
....
....
....

Date:................................

Weight:.......................

NUTRITION

Number of Meals............

Protein	YES/NO
Fruit & vegetables	YES/NO
Healthy Fat	YES/NO
Fibre	YES/NO
Apple Cider Vinegar	YES/NO
Supplements	YES/NO

METABOLISM

Cold Exposure   YES/NO

Aerobic Exercise

✓   ....
✓   ....

Anaerobic Exercise

✓   ....
✓   ....
✓   ....
✓   ....
✓   ....
✓   ....
✓   ....

Flexibility Exercise

✓   ....
✓   ....

TIMING

A Good Night's Sleep YES/NO

Breakfast...........................

Dinner Completed..............

Window..........................

Digital Curfew...................

Bedtime...........................

MINDSET

Relaxation
....
....

Mindful Eating   YES/NO

Gratitude
....
....
....

Self-care & Kindness
....
....

Visualisation   YES/NO

Creativity/Joy/Fun
....
....

Connection/Love
....
....

Priorities/Focus/Purpose
....
....
....
....

Date:...........................

Weight:......................

NUTRITION

Number of Meals............

Protein	YES/NO
Fruit & vegetables	YES/NO
Healthy Fat	YES/NO
Fibre	YES/NO
Apple Cider Vinegar	YES/NO
Supplements	YES/NO

METABOLISM

Cold Exposure   YES/NO

Aerobic Exercise
 ✓ ....
 ✓ ....

Anaerobic Exercise
 ✓ ....
 ✓ ....
 ✓ ....
 ✓ ....
 ✓ ....
 ✓ ....
 ✓ ....

Flexibility Exercise
 ✓ ....
 ✓ ....

WEEKLY REVIEW

Weight:

Review.............................

Weight:

Focus.............................

TIMING:

Review...............................
....
....
....
....

TIMING:

Focus...............................
....
....
....
....

MINDSET:

Review...............................
....
....
....
....
....
....

MINDSET:

Focus...............................
....
....
....
....
....
....

NUTRITION:

Review ....
....
....
....
....
....

NUTRITION:

Focus...............................
....
....
....
....
....

METABOLISM:

Review...............................
....
....
....
....

METABOLISM:

Focus...............................
....
....
....
....

"In the depth of winter I finally learned that there was in me an invincible summer."

Albert Camus

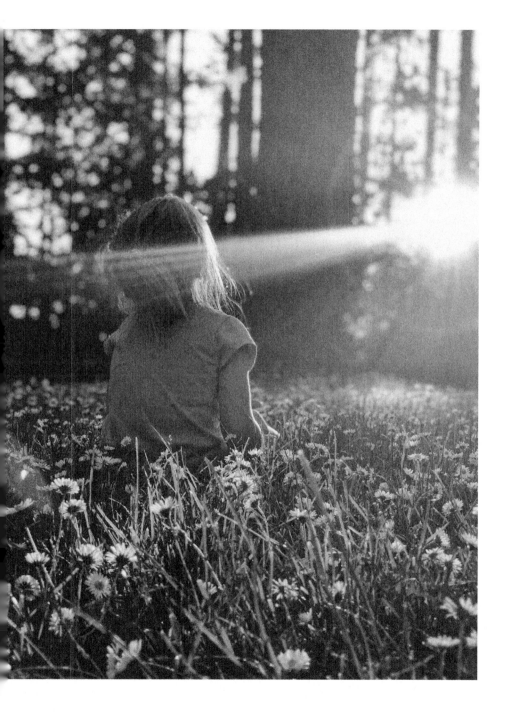

TIMING

A Good Night's Sleep YES/NO

Breakfast...........................

Dinner Completed..............

Window.........................

Digital Curfew...................

Bedtime..........................

MINDSET

Relaxation

....

....

Mindful Eating   YES/NO

Gratitude

....

....

....

Self-care & Kindness

....

....

Visualisation   YES/NO

Creativity/Joy/Fun

....

....

Connection/Love

....

....

Priorities/Focus/Purpose

....

....

....

....

Date:................................

Weight:.....................

NUTRITION

Number of Meals............

Protein	YES/NO
Fruit & vegetables	YES/NO
Healthy Fat	YES/NO
Fibre	YES/NO
Apple Cider Vinegar	YES/NO
Supplements	YES/NO

METABOLISM

Cold Exposure   YES/NO

Aerobic Exercise

✓ ....

✓ ....

Anaerobic Exercise

✓ ....

✓ ....

✓ ....

✓ ....

✓ ....

✓ ....

✓ ....

Flexibility Exercise

✓ ....

✓ ....

TIMING

A Good Night's Sleep YES/NO

Breakfast..............................

Dinner Completed...............

Window............................

Digital Curfew...................

Bedtime............................

MINDSET

Relaxation

....
....

Mindful Eating   YES/NO

Gratitude

....
....
....

Self-care & Kindness

....
....

Visualisation   YES/NO

Creativity/Joy/Fun

....
....

Connection/Love

....
....

Priorities/Focus/Purpose

....
....
....
....

Date:.................................

Weight:.......................

NUTRITION

Number of Meals.............

Protein   YES/NO

Fruit & vegetables   YES/NO

Healthy Fat   YES/NO

Fibre   YES/NO

Apple Cider Vinegar   YES/NO

Supplements   YES/NO

METABOLISM

Cold Exposure   YES/NO

Aerobic Exercise

✓   ....
✓   ....

Anaerobic Exercise

✓   ....
✓   ....
✓   ....
✓   ....
✓   ....
✓   ....
✓   ....

Flexibility Exercise

✓   ....
✓   ....

TIMING

A Good Night's Sleep YES/NO

Breakfast............................

Dinner Completed...............

Window............................

Digital Curfew...................

Bedtime............................

MINDSET

Relaxation

....
....

Mindful Eating   YES/NO

Gratitude

....
....
....

Self-care & Kindness

....
....

Visualisation   YES/NO

Creativity/Joy/Fun

....
....

Connection/Love

....
....

Priorities/Focus/Purpose

....
....
....
....

Date:...................................

Weight:.....................

NUTRITION

Number of Meals............

Protein   YES/NO

Fruit & vegetables   YES/NO

Healthy Fat   YES/NO

Fibre   YES/NO

Apple Cider Vinegar   YES/NO

Supplements   YES/NO

METABOLISM

Cold Exposure   YES/NO

Aerobic Exercise

✓ ....
✓ ....

Anaerobic Exercise

✓ ....
✓ ....
✓ ....
✓ ....
✓ ....
✓ ....
✓ ....

Flexibility Exercise

✓ ....
✓ ....

TIMING

A Good Night's Sleep YES/NO

Breakfast...........................

Dinner Completed...............

Window...........................

Digital Curfew...................

Bedtime...........................

MINDSET

Relaxation

....
....

Mindful Eating   YES/NO

Gratitude

....
....
....

Self-care & Kindness

....
....

Visualisation   YES/NO

Creativity/Joy/Fun

....
....

Connection/Love

....
....

Priorities/Focus/Purpose

....
....
....
....

Date:.................................

Weight:.......................

NUTRITION

Number of Meals.............

Protein	YES/NO
Fruit & vegetables	YES/NO
Healthy Fat	YES/NO
Fibre	YES/NO
Apple Cider Vinegar	YES/NO
Supplements	YES/NO

METABOLISM

Cold Exposure   YES/NO

Aerobic Exercise

✓ ....
✓ ....

Anaerobic Exercise

✓ ....
✓ ....
✓ ....
✓ ....
✓ ....
✓ ....
✓ ....

Flexibility Exercise

✓ ....
✓ ....

TIMING

A Good Night's Sleep YES/NO

Breakfast...........................

Dinner Completed...............

Window..........................

Digital Curfew...................

Bedtime..........................

MINDSET

Relaxation

....
....

Mindful Eating   YES/NO

Gratitude

....
....
....

Self-care & Kindness

....
....

Visualisation   YES/NO

Creativity/Joy/Fun

....
....

Connection/Love

....
....

Priorities/Focus/Purpose

....
....
....
....

Date:...............................

Weight:......................

NUTRITION

Number of Meals............

Protein   YES/NO

Fruit & vegetables   YES/NO

Healthy Fat   YES/NO

Fibre   YES/NO

Apple Cider Vinegar   YES/NO

Supplements   YES/NO

METABOLISM

Cold Exposure   YES/NO

Aerobic Exercise

   ✓ ....
   ✓ ....

Anaerobic Exercise

   ✓ ....
   ✓ ....
   ✓ ....
   ✓ ....
   ✓ ....
   ✓ ....
   ✓ ....

Flexibility Exercise

   ✓ ....
   ✓ ....

TIMING

A Good Night's Sleep YES/NO

Breakfast............................

Dinner Completed................

Window...........................

Digital Curfew....................

Bedtime...........................

MINDSET

Relaxation

....

....

Mindful Eating   YES/NO

Gratitude

....

....

....

Self-care & Kindness

....

....

Visualisation   YES/NO

Creativity/Joy/Fun

....

....

Connection/Love

....

....

Priorities/Focus/Purpose

....

....

....

....

Date:................................

Weight:......................

NUTRITION

Number of Meals............

Protein	YES/NO
Fruit & vegetables	YES/NO
Healthy Fat	YES/NO
Fibre	YES/NO
Apple Cider Vinegar	YES/NO
Supplements	YES/NO

METABOLISM

Cold Exposure   YES/NO

Aerobic Exercise

✓   ....

✓   ....

Anaerobic Exercise

✓   ....

✓   ....

✓   ....

✓   ....

✓   ....

✓   ....

✓   ....

Flexibility Exercise

✓   ....

✓   ....

TIMING

A Good Night's Sleep YES/NO

Breakfast...........................

Dinner Completed...............

Window............................

Digital Curfew...................

Bedtime............................

MINDSET

Relaxation

....
....

Mindful Eating   YES/NO

Gratitude

....
....
....

Self-care & Kindness

....
....

Visualisation   YES/NO

Creativity/Joy/Fun

....
....

Connection/Love

....
....

Priorities/Focus/Purpose

....
....
....
....

Date:................................

Weight:.......................

NUTRITION

Number of Meals............

Protein	YES/NO
Fruit & vegetables	YES/NO
Healthy Fat	YES/NO
Fibre	YES/NO
Apple Cider Vinegar	YES/NO
Supplements	YES/NO

METABOLISM

Cold Exposure   YES/NO

Aerobic Exercise

✓ ....
✓ ....

Anaerobic Exercise

✓ ....
✓ ....
✓ ....
✓ ....
✓ ....
✓ ....
✓ ....

Flexibility Exercise

✓ ....
✓ ....

WEEKLY REVIEW

Weight:

Review.............................

Weight:

Focus.............................

TIMING:

Review.............................
....
....
....
....

TIMING:

Focus.............................
....
....
....
....

MINDSET:

Review.............................
....
....
....
....
....
....

MINDSET:

Focus.............................
....
....
....
....
....
....

NUTRITION:

Review ....
....
....
....
....
....

NUTRITION:

Focus.............................
....
....
....
....
....

METABOLISM:

Review.............................
....
....
....
....

METABOLISM:

Focus.............................
....
....
....
....

"Optimism is the faith that leads to achievement. Nothing can be done without hope and confidence."

Helen Keller

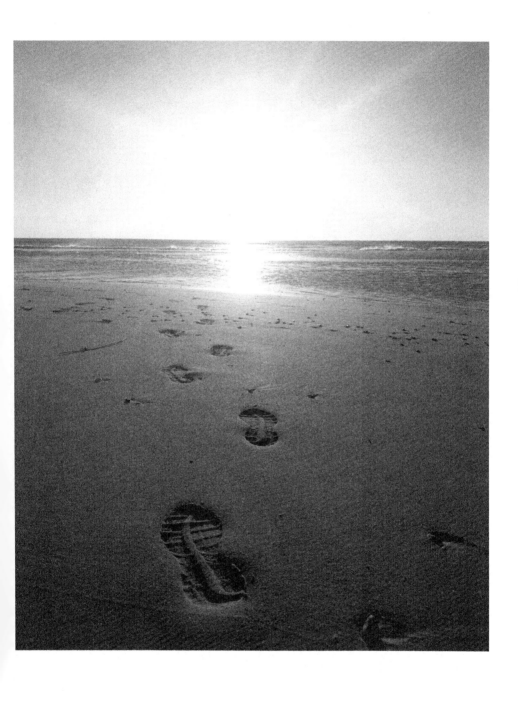

TIMING

A Good Night's Sleep YES/NO

Breakfast...........................

Dinner Completed...............

Window............................

Digital Curfew...................

Bedtime............................

MINDSET

Relaxation

....
....

Mindful Eating   YES/NO

Gratitude

....
....
....

Self-care & Kindness

....
....

Visualisation   YES/NO

Creativity/Joy/Fun

....
....

Connection/Love

....
....

Priorities/Focus/Purpose

....
....
....
....

Date:...............................

Weight:........................

NUTRITION

Number of Meals.............

Protein   YES/NO

Fruit & vegetables   YES/NO

Healthy Fat   YES/NO

Fibre   YES/NO

Apple Cider Vinegar   YES/NO

Supplements   YES/NO

METABOLISM

Cold Exposure   YES/NO

Aerobic Exercise

✓   ....
✓   ....

Anaerobic Exercise

✓   ....
✓   ....
✓   ....
✓   ....
✓   ....
✓   ....
✓   ....

Flexibility Exercise

✓   ....
✓   ....

TIMING

A Good Night's Sleep YES/NO

Breakfast...........................

Dinner Completed...............

Window...........................

Digital Curfew...................

Bedtime...........................

MINDSET

Relaxation

....

....

Mindful Eating   YES/NO

Gratitude

....

....

....

Self-care & Kindness

....

....

Visualisation   YES/NO

Creativity/Joy/Fun

....

....

Connection/Love

....

....

Priorities/Focus/Purpose

....

....

....

....

Date:...............................

Weight:.......................

NUTRITION

Number of Meals............

Protein	YES/NO
Fruit & vegetables	YES/NO
Healthy Fat	YES/NO
Fibre	YES/NO
Apple Cider Vinegar	YES/NO
Supplements	YES/NO

METABOLISM

Cold Exposure   YES/NO

Aerobic Exercise

✓   ....

✓   ....

Anaerobic Exercise

✓   ....

✓   ....

✓   ....

✓   ....

✓   ....

✓   ....

✓   ....

Flexibility Exercise

✓   ....

✓   ....

TIMING

A Good Night's Sleep YES/NO

Breakfast...........................

Dinner Completed...............

Window...........................

Digital Curfew...................

Bedtime...........................

Date:................................

Weight:........................

NUTRITION

Number of Meals............

Protein	YES/NO
Fruit & vegetables	YES/NO
Healthy Fat	YES/NO
Fibre	YES/NO
Apple Cider Vinegar	YES/NO
Supplements	YES/NO

MINDSET

Relaxation

....

....

Mindful Eating   YES/NO

Gratitude

....

....

....

Self-care & Kindness

....

....

Visualisation   YES/NO

Creativity/Joy/Fun

....

....

Connection/Love

....

....

Priorities/Focus/Purpose

....

....

....

....

METABOLISM

Cold Exposure   YES/NO

Aerobic Exercise

✓ ....

✓ ....

Anaerobic Exercise

✓ ....

✓ ....

✓ ....

✓ ....

✓ ....

✓ ....

✓ ....

Flexibility Exercise

✓ ....

✓ ....

TIMING

A Good Night's Sleep YES/NO

Breakfast..............................

Dinner Completed...............

Window..........................

Digital Curfew...................

Bedtime...........................

MINDSET

Relaxation

....

....

Mindful Eating   YES/NO

Gratitude

....

....

....

Self-care & Kindness

....

....

Visualisation   YES/NO

Creativity/Joy/Fun

....

....

Connection/Love

....

....

Priorities/Focus/Purpose

....

....

....

....

Date:................................

Weight:.......................

NUTRITION

Number of Meals............

Protein	YES/NO
Fruit & vegetables	YES/NO
Healthy Fat	YES/NO
Fibre	YES/NO
Apple Cider Vinegar	YES/NO
Supplements	YES/NO

METABOLISM

Cold Exposure   YES/NO

Aerobic Exercise

✓ ....

✓ ....

Anaerobic Exercise

✓ ....

✓ ....

✓ ....

✓ ....

✓ ....

✓ ....

✓ ....

Flexibility Exercise

✓ ....

✓ ....

TIMING

A Good Night's Sleep YES/NO

Breakfast...........................

Dinner Completed...............

Window..........................

Digital Curfew...................

Bedtime...........................

MINDSET

Relaxation

....

....

Mindful Eating   YES/NO

Gratitude

....

....

....

Self-care & Kindness

....

....

Visualisation   YES/NO

Creativity/Joy/Fun

....

....

Connection/Love

....

....

Priorities/Focus/Purpose

....

....

....

....

Date:.................................

Weight:......................

NUTRITION

Number of Meals.............

Protein	YES/NO
Fruit & vegetables	YES/NO
Healthy Fat	YES/NO
Fibre	YES/NO
Apple Cider Vinegar	YES/NO
Supplements	YES/NO

METABOLISM

Cold Exposure   YES/NO

Aerobic Exercise

✓ ....

✓ ....

Anaerobic Exercise

✓ ....

✓ ....

✓ ....

✓ ....

✓ ....

✓ ....

✓ ....

Flexibility Exercise

✓ ....

✓ ....

TIMING

A Good Night's Sleep YES/NO

Breakfast...........................

Dinner Completed...............

Window...........................

Digital Curfew...................

Bedtime...........................

MINDSET

Relaxation

....
....

Mindful Eating   YES/NO

Gratitude

....
....
....

Self-care & Kindness

....
....

Visualisation   YES/NO

Creativity/Joy/Fun

....
....

Connection/Love

....
....

Priorities/Focus/Purpose

....
....
....
....

Date:...............................

Weight:.......................

NUTRITION

Number of Meals............

Protein	YES/NO
Fruit & vegetables	YES/NO
Healthy Fat	YES/NO
Fibre	YES/NO
Apple Cider Vinegar	YES/NO
Supplements	YES/NO

METABOLISM

Cold Exposure   YES/NO

Aerobic Exercise

✓ ....
✓ ....

Anaerobic Exercise

✓ ....
✓ ....
✓ ....
✓ ....
✓ ....
✓ ....
✓ ....

Flexibility Exercise

✓ ....
✓ ....

TIMING

A Good Night's Sleep YES/NO

Breakfast.............................

Dinner Completed...............

Window............................

Digital Curfew....................

Bedtime............................

MINDSET

Relaxation

....
....

Mindful Eating   YES/NO

Gratitude

....
....
....

Self-care & Kindness

....
....

Visualisation   YES/NO

Creativity/Joy/Fun

....
....

Connection/Love

....
....

Priorities/Focus/Purpose

....
....
....
....

Date:.................................

Weight:.......................

NUTRITION

Number of Meals............

Protein   YES/NO

Fruit & vegetables   YES/NO

Healthy Fat   YES/NO

Fibre   YES/NO

Apple Cider Vinegar   YES/NO

Supplements   YES/NO

METABOLISM

Cold Exposure   YES/NO

Aerobic Exercise

✓   ....
✓   ....

Anaerobic Exercise

✓   ....
✓   ....
✓   ....
✓   ....
✓   ....
✓   ....
✓   ....

Flexibility Exercise

✓   ....
✓   ....

WEEKLY REVIEW

Weight:

Review.............................

Weight:

Focus.................................

TIMING:

Review................................
....
....
....
....

TIMING:

Focus...............................
....
....
....
....

MINDSET:

Review................................
....
....
....
....
....
....

MINDSET:

Focus..................................
....
....
....
....
....
....

NUTRITION:

Review ....
....
....
....
....
....

NUTRITION:

Focus...............................
....
....
....
....
....

METABOLISM:

Review................................
....
....
....
....

METABOLISM:

Focus...............................
....
....
....
....

"My mission in life is not merely to survive, but to thrive; and to do so with some passion, some compassion, some humour, and some style."

Maya Angelou

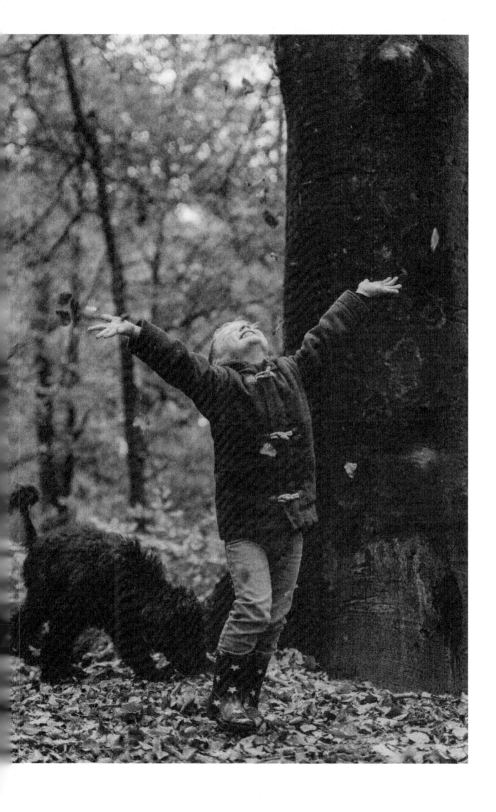

TIMING

A Good Night's Sleep YES/NO

Breakfast...........................

Dinner Completed...............

Window...........................

Digital Curfew...................

Bedtime...........................

MINDSET

Relaxation
....
....

Mindful Eating YES/NO

Gratitude
....
....
....

Self-care & Kindness
....
....

Visualisation YES/NO

Creativity/Joy/Fun
....
....

Connection/Love
....
....

Priorities/Focus/Purpose
....
....
....
....

Date:...............................

Weight:......................

NUTRITION

Number of Meals............

Protein	YES/NO
Fruit & vegetables	YES/NO
Healthy Fat	YES/NO
Fibre	YES/NO
Apple Cider Vinegar	YES/NO
Supplements	YES/NO

METABOLISM

Cold Exposure YES/NO

Aerobic Exercise
- ✓ ....
- ✓ ....

Anaerobic Exercise
- ✓ ....
- ✓ ....
- ✓ ....
- ✓ ....
- ✓ ....
- ✓ ....
- ✓ ....

Flexibility Exercise
- ✓ ....
- ✓ ....

TIMING

A Good Night's Sleep YES/NO

Breakfast...........................

Dinner Completed...............

Window............................

Digital Curfew...................

Bedtime...........................

MINDSET

Relaxation
....
....

Mindful Eating   YES/NO

Gratitude
....
....
....

Self-care & Kindness
....
....

Visualisation   YES/NO

Creativity/Joy/Fun
....
....

Connection/Love
....
....

Priorities/Focus/Purpose
....
....
....
....

Date:................................

Weight:.....................

NUTRITION

Number of Meals............

Protein	YES/NO
Fruit & vegetables	YES/NO
Healthy Fat	YES/NO
Fibre	YES/NO
Apple Cider Vinegar	YES/NO
Supplements	YES/NO

METABOLISM

Cold Exposure   YES/NO

Aerobic Exercise

✓ ....
✓ ....

Anaerobic Exercise

✓ ....
✓ ....
✓ ....
✓ ....
✓ ....
✓ ....
✓ ....

Flexibility Exercise

✓ ....
✓ ....

TIMING

A Good Night's Sleep YES/NO

Breakfast............................

Dinner Completed...............

Window...........................

Digital Curfew...................

Bedtime...........................

MINDSET

Relaxation
....
....

Mindful Eating   YES/NO

Gratitude
....
....
....

Self-care & Kindness
....
....

Visualisation   YES/NO

Creativity/Joy/Fun
....
....

Connection/Love
....
....

Priorities/Focus/Purpose
....
....
....
....

Date:................................

Weight:........................

NUTRITION

Number of Meals.............

Protein   YES/NO

Fruit & vegetables   YES/NO

Healthy Fat   YES/NO

Fibre   YES/NO

Apple Cider Vinegar   YES/NO

Supplements   YES/NO

METABOLISM

Cold Exposure   YES/NO

Aerobic Exercise
   ✓ ....
   ✓ ....

Anaerobic Exercise
   ✓ ....
   ✓ ....
   ✓ ....
   ✓ ....
   ✓ ....
   ✓ ....
   ✓ ....

Flexibility Exercise
   ✓ ....
   ✓ ....

TIMING

A Good Night's Sleep YES/NO

Breakfast...........................

Dinner Completed...............

Window...........................

Digital Curfew...................

Bedtime...........................

MINDSET

Relaxation

....
....

Mindful Eating   YES/NO

Gratitude

....
....
....

Self-care & Kindness

....
....

Visualisation   YES/NO

Creativity/Joy/Fun

....
....

Connection/Love

....
....

Priorities/Focus/Purpose

....
....
....
....

Date:...............................

Weight:.......................

NUTRITION

Number of Meals............

Protein	YES/NO
Fruit & vegetables	YES/NO
Healthy Fat	YES/NO
Fibre	YES/NO
Apple Cider Vinegar	YES/NO
Supplements	YES/NO

METABOLISM

Cold Exposure   YES/NO

Aerobic Exercise

✓ ....
✓ ....

Anaerobic Exercise

✓ ....
✓ ....
✓ ....
✓ ....
✓ ....
✓ ....
✓ ....

Flexibility Exercise

✓ ....
✓ ....

TIMING

A Good Night's Sleep YES/NO

Breakfast...........................

Dinner Completed..............

Window..........................

Digital Curfew...................

Bedtime..........................

MINDSET

Relaxation

....

....

Mindful Eating   YES/NO

Gratitude

....

....

....

Self-care & Kindness

....

....

Visualisation   YES/NO

Creativity/Joy/Fun

....

....

Connection/Love

....

....

Priorities/Focus/Purpose

....

....

....

....

Date:................................

Weight:.......................

NUTRITION

Number of Meals............

Protein	YES/NO
Fruit & vegetables	YES/NO
Healthy Fat	YES/NO
Fibre	YES/NO
Apple Cider Vinegar	YES/NO
Supplements	YES/NO

METABOLISM

Cold Exposure   YES/NO

Aerobic Exercise

✓   ....

✓   ....

Anaerobic Exercise

✓   ....

✓   ....

✓   ....

✓   ....

✓   ....

✓   ....

✓   ....

Flexibility Exercise

✓   ....

✓   ....

TIMING

A Good Night's Sleep YES/NO

Breakfast...........................

Dinner Completed...............

Window...........................

Digital Curfew...................

Bedtime...........................

MINDSET

Relaxation

....

....

Mindful Eating   YES/NO

Gratitude

....

....

....

Self-care & Kindness

....

....

Visualisation   YES/NO

Creativity/Joy/Fun

....

....

Connection/Love

....

....

Priorities/Focus/Purpose

....

....

....

....

Date:...............................

Weight:.......................

NUTRITION

Number of Meals............

Protein	YES/NO
Fruit & vegetables	YES/NO
Healthy Fat	YES/NO
Fibre	YES/NO
Apple Cider Vinegar	YES/NO
Supplements	YES/NO

METABOLISM

Cold Exposure   YES/NO

Aerobic Exercise

✓   ....
✓   ....

Anaerobic Exercise

✓   ....
✓   ....
✓   ....
✓   ....
✓   ....
✓   ....
✓   ....

Flexibility Exercise

✓   ....
✓   ....

TIMING

A Good Night's Sleep YES/NO

Breakfast...........................

Dinner Completed...............

Window...........................

Digital Curfew...................

Bedtime...........................

MINDSET

Relaxation

....

....

Mindful Eating   YES/NO

Gratitude

....

....

....

Self-care & Kindness

....

....

Visualisation   YES/NO

Creativity/Joy/Fun

....

....

Connection/Love

....

....

Priorities/Focus/Purpose

....

....

....

....

Date:................................

Weight:.......................

NUTRITION

Number of Meals............

Protein   YES/NO

Fruit & vegetables   YES/NO

Healthy Fat   YES/NO

Fibre   YES/NO

Apple Cider Vinegar   YES/NO

Supplements   YES/NO

METABOLISM

Cold Exposure   YES/NO

Aerobic Exercise

✓   ....

✓   ....

Anaerobic Exercise

✓   ....

✓   ....

✓   ....

✓   ....

✓   ....

✓   ....

✓   ....

Flexibility Exercise

✓   ....

✓   ....

WEEKLY REVIEW

Weight:

Review............................

Weight:

Focus............................

TIMING:

Review............................
....
....
....
....

TIMING:

Focus............................
....
....
....
....

MINDSET:

Review............................
....
....
....
....
....
....

MINDSET:

Focus............................
....
....
....
....
....
....

NUTRITION:

Review ....
....
....
....
....

NUTRITION:

Focus............................
....
....
....
....

METABOLISM:

Review............................
....
....
....

METABOLISM:

Focus............................
....
....
....

WEEK EIGHT

"Our greatest weakness lies in giving up. The most certain way to succeed is always to try just one more time."

Thomas A. Edison

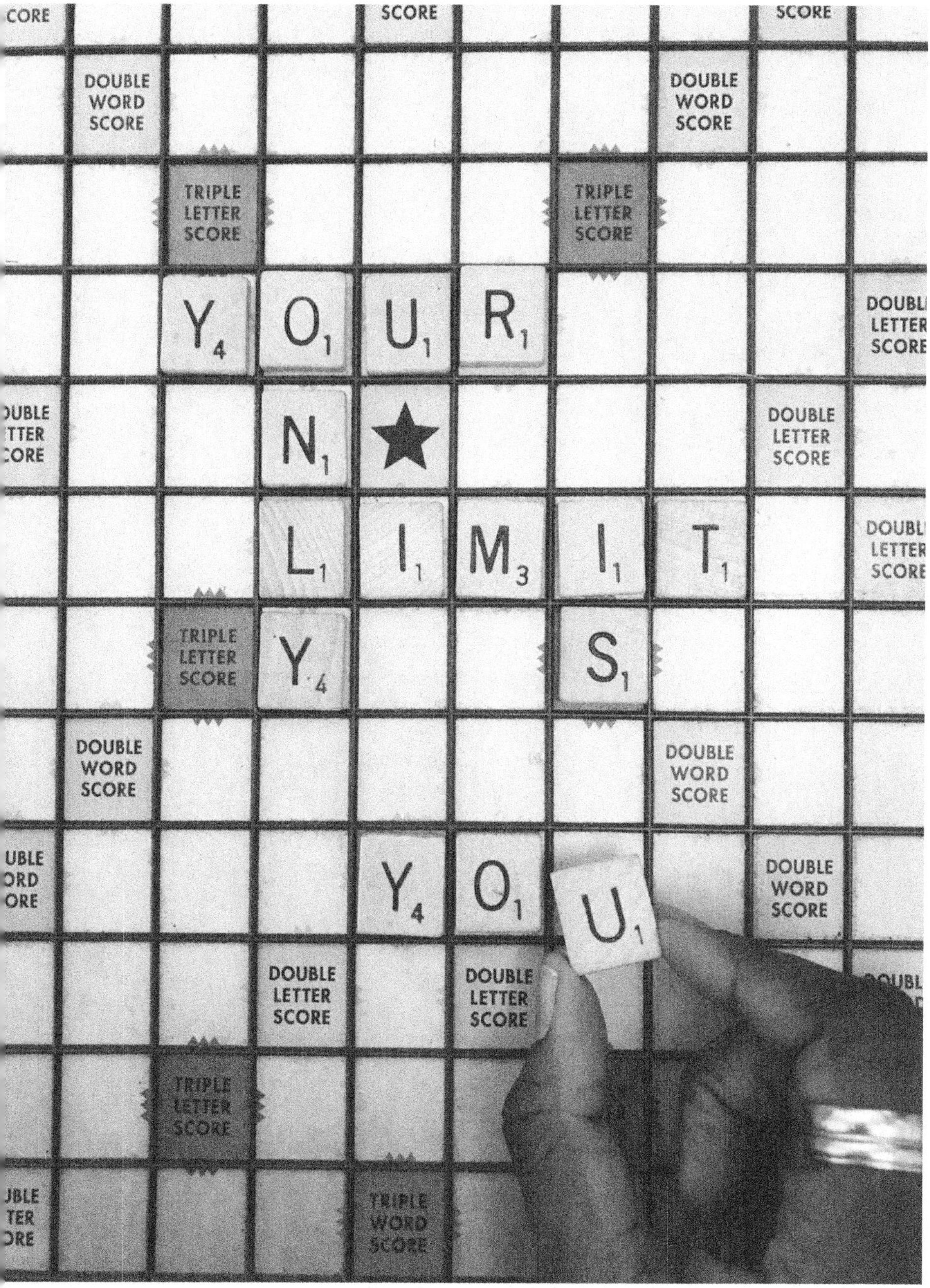
YOUR
ONLY
LIMIT
IS
YOU
DOUBLE WORD SCORE
TRIPLE LETTER SCORE
DOUBLE LETTER SCORE
TRIPLE WORD SCORE

TIMING

A Good Night's Sleep YES/NO

Breakfast...........................

Dinner Completed...............

Window............................

Digital Curfew...................

Bedtime............................

MINDSET

Relaxation

....

....

Mindful Eating   YES/NO

Gratitude

....

....

....

Self-care & Kindness

....

....

Visualisation   YES/NO

Creativity/Joy/Fun

....

....

Connection/Love

....

....

Priorities/Focus/Purpose

....

....

....

....

Date:................................

Weight:.....................

NUTRITION

Number of Meals............

Protein	YES/NO
Fruit & vegetables	YES/NO
Healthy Fat	YES/NO
Fibre	YES/NO
Apple Cider Vinegar	YES/NO
Supplements	YES/NO

METABOLISM

Cold Exposure   YES/NO

Aerobic Exercise

  ✓ ....

  ✓ ....

Anaerobic Exercise

  ✓ ....

  ✓ ....

  ✓ ....

  ✓ ....

  ✓ ....

  ✓ ....

  ✓ ....

Flexibility Exercise

  ✓ ....

  ✓ ....

TIMING

A Good Night's Sleep YES/NO

Breakfast..........................

Dinner Completed...............

Window...........................

Digital Curfew...................

Bedtime...........................

MINDSET

Relaxation
....
....

Mindful Eating   YES/NO

Gratitude
....
....
....

Self-care & Kindness
....
....

Visualisation   YES/NO

Creativity/Joy/Fun
....
....

Connection/Love
....
....

Priorities/Focus/Purpose
....
....
....
....

Date:.............................

Weight:........................

NUTRITION

Number of Meals............

Protein   YES/NO

Fruit & vegetables   YES/NO

Healthy Fat   YES/NO

Fibre   YES/NO

Apple Cider Vinegar   YES/NO

Supplements   YES/NO

METABOLISM

Cold Exposure   YES/NO

Aerobic Exercise
✓   ....
✓   ....

Anaerobic Exercise
✓   ....
✓   ....
✓   ....
✓   ....
✓   ....
✓   ....
✓   ....

Flexibility Exercise
✓   ....
✓   ....

TIMING

A Good Night's Sleep YES/NO

Breakfast...........................

Dinner Completed...............

Window...........................

Digital Curfew...................

Bedtime...........................

MINDSET

Relaxation

....
....

Mindful Eating   YES/NO

Gratitude

....
....
....

Self-care & Kindness

....
....

Visualisation   YES/NO

Creativity/Joy/Fun

....
....

Connection/Love

....
....

Priorities/Focus/Purpose

....
....
....
....

Date:.............................

Weight:........................

NUTRITION

Number of Meals............

Protein	YES/NO
Fruit & vegetables	YES/NO
Healthy Fat	YES/NO
Fibre	YES/NO
Apple Cider Vinegar	YES/NO
Supplements	YES/NO

METABOLISM

Cold Exposure   YES/NO

Aerobic Exercise

✓ ....
✓ ....

Anaerobic Exercise

✓ ....
✓ ....
✓ ....
✓ ....
✓ ....
✓ ....
✓ ....

Flexibility Exercise

✓ ....
✓ ....

TIMING

A Good Night's Sleep YES/NO

Breakfast...........................

Dinner Completed...............

Window...........................

Digital Curfew...................

Bedtime...........................

Date:................................

Weight:......................

NUTRITION

Number of Meals............

Protein	YES/NO
Fruit & vegetables	YES/NO
Healthy Fat	YES/NO
Fibre	YES/NO
Apple Cider Vinegar	YES/NO
Supplements	YES/NO

MINDSET

Relaxation

....
....

Mindful Eating   YES/NO

Gratitude

....
....
....

Self-care & Kindness

....
....

Visualisation   YES/NO

Creativity/Joy/Fun

....
....

Connection/Love

....
....

Priorities/Focus/Purpose

....
....
....
....

METABOLISM

Cold Exposure   YES/NO

Aerobic Exercise

✓ ....
✓ ....

Anaerobic Exercise

✓ ....
✓ ....
✓ ....
✓ ....
✓ ....
✓ ....
✓ ....

Flexibility Exercise

✓ ....
✓ ....

TIMING

A Good Night's Sleep YES/NO

Breakfast...........................

Dinner Completed..............

Window...........................

Digital Curfew...................

Bedtime...........................

MINDSET

Relaxation

....
....

Mindful Eating   YES/NO

Gratitude

....
....
....

Self-care & Kindness

....
....

Visualisation   YES/NO

Creativity/Joy/Fun

....
....

Connection/Love

....
....

Priorities/Focus/Purpose

....
....
....
....

Date:.................................

Weight:......................

NUTRITION

Number of Meals............

Protein	YES/NO
Fruit & vegetables	YES/NO
Healthy Fat	YES/NO
Fibre	YES/NO
Apple Cider Vinegar	YES/NO
Supplements	YES/NO

METABOLISM

Cold Exposure   YES/NO

Aerobic Exercise

✓   ....
✓   ....

Anaerobic Exercise

✓   ....
✓   ....
✓   ....
✓   ....
✓   ....
✓   ....
✓   ....

Flexibility Exercise

✓   ....
✓   ....

TIMING

A Good Night's Sleep YES/NO

Breakfast...........................

Dinner Completed..............

Window...........................

Digital Curfew..................

Bedtime..........................

MINDSET

Relaxation

....

....

Mindful Eating   YES/NO

Gratitude

....

....

....

Self-care & Kindness

....

....

Visualisation   YES/NO

Creativity/Joy/Fun

....

....

Connection/Love

....

....

Priorities/Focus/Purpose

....

....

....

....

Date:...............................

Weight:.......................

NUTRITION

Number of Meals............

Protein	YES/NO
Fruit & vegetables	YES/NO
Healthy Fat	YES/NO
Fibre	YES/NO
Apple Cider Vinegar	YES/NO
Supplements	YES/NO

METABOLISM

Cold Exposure   YES/NO

Aerobic Exercise

✓   ....

✓   ....

Anaerobic Exercise

✓   ....

✓   ....

✓   ....

✓   ....

✓   ....

✓   ....

✓   ....

Flexibility Exercise

✓   ....

✓   ....

TIMING

A Good Night's Sleep YES/NO

Breakfast...........................

Dinner Completed..............

Window...........................

Digital Curfew...................

Bedtime...........................

MINDSET

Relaxation
....
....

Mindful Eating   YES/NO

Gratitude
....
....
....

Self-care & Kindness
....
....

Visualisation   YES/NO

Creativity/Joy/Fun
....
....

Connection/Love
....
....

Priorities/Focus/Purpose
....
....
....
....

Date:..............................

Weight:......................

NUTRITION

Number of Meals.............

Protein	YES/NO
Fruit & vegetables	YES/NO
Healthy Fat	YES/NO
Fibre	YES/NO
Apple Cider Vinegar	YES/NO
Supplements	YES/NO

METABOLISM

Cold Exposure   YES/NO

Aerobic Exercise

✓   ....
✓   ....

Anaerobic Exercise

✓   ....
✓   ....
✓   ....
✓   ....
✓   ....
✓   ....
✓   ....

Flexibility Exercise

✓   ....
✓   ....

WEEKLY REVIEW

Weight:

Review............................

TIMING:

Review................................
....
....
....
....

MINDSET:

Review................................
....
....
....
....
....
....

NUTRITION:

Review ....
....
....
....
....
....

METABOLISM:

Review................................
....
....
....

Weight:

Focus..............................

TIMING:

Focus................................
....
....
....
....

MINDSET:

Focus................................
....
....
....
....
....
....

NUTRITION:

Focus................................
....
....
....
....
....

METABOLISM:

Focus................................
....
....
....

"Either you run the day or the day runs you."

Jim Rohn

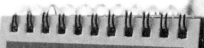

Life is short.
Do stuff
that matters

SEP	S	M	T	W	T	F	S
18	30						
	2	3	4	5	6	7	1
	9	10	11	12	13	14	8
	16	17	18	19	20	21	15
	23	24	25	26	27	28	22
							29

TIMING

A Good Night's Sleep YES/NO

Breakfast...........................

Dinner Completed...............

Window...........................

Digital Curfew...................

Bedtime...........................

MINDSET

Relaxation
....
....

Mindful Eating   YES/NO

Gratitude
....
....
....

Self-care & Kindness
....
....

Visualisation   YES/NO

Creativity/Joy/Fun
....
....

Connection/Love
....
....

Priorities/Focus/Purpose
....
....
....
....

Date:..

Weight:........................

NUTRITION

Number of Meals.............

Protein	YES/NO
Fruit & vegetables	YES/NO
Healthy Fat	YES/NO
Fibre	YES/NO
Apple Cider Vinegar	YES/NO
Supplements	YES/NO

METABOLISM

Cold Exposure   YES/NO

Aerobic Exercise
- ✓ ....
- ✓ ....,,

Anaerobic Exercise
- ✓ ....
- ✓ ....
- ✓ ....
- ✓ ....
- ✓ ....
- ✓ ....
- ✓ ....

Flexibility Exercise
- ✓ ....
- ✓ ....

TIMING

A Good Night's Sleep YES/NO

Breakfast...........................

Dinner Completed..............

Window...........................

Digital Curfew...................

Bedtime...........................

MINDSET

Relaxation

....

....

Mindful Eating   YES/NO

Gratitude

....

....

....

Self-care & Kindness

....

....

Visualisation   YES/NO

Creativity/Joy/Fun

....

....

Connection/Love

....

....

Priorities/Focus/Purpose

....

....

....

....

Date:................................

Weight:......................

NUTRITION

Number of Meals............

Protein	YES/NO
Fruit & vegetables	YES/NO
Healthy Fat	YES/NO
Fibre	YES/NO
Apple Cider Vinegar	YES/NO
Supplements	YES/NO

METABOLISM

Cold Exposure   YES/NO

Aerobic Exercise

✓   ....

✓   ....

Anaerobic Exercise

✓   ....

✓   ....

✓   ....

✓   ....

✓   ....

✓   ....

✓   ....

Flexibility Exercise

✓   ....

✓   ....

TIMING

A Good Night's Sleep YES/NO

Breakfast...........................

Dinner Completed...............

Window...........................

Digital Curfew...................

Bedtime...........................

MINDSET

Relaxation

....

....

Mindful Eating   YES/NO

Gratitude

....

....

....

Self-care & Kindness

....

....

Visualisation   YES/NO

Creativity/Joy/Fun

....

....

Connection/Love

....

....

Priorities/Focus/Purpose

....

....

....

....

Date:................................

Weight:.......................

NUTRITION

Number of Meals............

Protein	YES/NO
Fruit & vegetables	YES/NO
Healthy Fat	YES/NO
Fibre	YES/NO
Apple Cider Vinegar	YES/NO
Supplements	YES/NO

METABOLISM

Cold Exposure   YES/NO

Aerobic Exercise

✓ ....

✓ ....

Anaerobic Exercise

✓ ....

✓ ....

✓ ....

✓ ....

✓ ....

✓ ....

✓ ....

Flexibility Exercise

✓ ....

✓ ....

TIMING

A Good Night's Sleep YES/NO

Breakfast...........................

Dinner Completed..............

Window..........................

Digital Curfew..................

Bedtime..........................

MINDSET

Relaxation

....
....

Mindful Eating   YES/NO

Gratitude

....
....
....

Self-care & Kindness

....
....

Visualisation   YES/NO

Creativity/Joy/Fun

....
....

Connection/Love

....
....

Priorities/Focus/Purpose

....
....
....
....

Date:...............................

Weight:......................

NUTRITION

Number of Meals............

Protein   YES/NO

Fruit & vegetables   YES/NO

Healthy Fat   YES/NO

Fibre   YES/NO

Apple Cider Vinegar   YES/NO

Supplements   YES/NO

METABOLISM

Cold Exposure   YES/NO

Aerobic Exercise

✓   ....
✓   ....

Anaerobic Exercise

✓   ....
✓   ....
✓   ....
✓   ....
✓   ....
✓   ....
✓   ....

Flexibility Exercise

✓   ....
✓   ....

TIMING

A Good Night's Sleep YES/NO

Breakfast...........................

Dinner Completed...............

Window...........................

Digital Curfew...................

Bedtime...........................

MINDSET

Relaxation
....
....

Mindful Eating   YES/NO

Gratitude
....
....
....

Self-care & Kindness
....
....

Visualisation   YES/NO

Creativity/Joy/Fun
....
....

Connection/Love
....
....

Priorities/Focus/Purpose
....
....
....
....

Date:................................

Weight:.....................

NUTRITION

Number of Meals............

Protein	YES/NO
Fruit & vegetables	YES/NO
Healthy Fat	YES/NO
Fibre	YES/NO
Apple Cider Vinegar	YES/NO
Supplements	YES/NO

METABOLISM

Cold Exposure   YES/NO

Aerobic Exercise
✓   ....
✓   ....

Anaerobic Exercise
✓   ....
✓   ....
✓   ....
✓   ....
✓   ....
✓   ....
✓   ....

Flexibility Exercise
✓   ....
✓   ....

TIMING

A Good Night's Sleep YES/NO

Breakfast...........................

Dinner Completed..............

Window..........................

Digital Curfew...................

Bedtime...........................

MINDSET

Relaxation

....
....

Mindful Eating   YES/NO

Gratitude

....
....
....

Self-care & Kindness

....
....

Visualisation   YES/NO

Creativity/Joy/Fun

....
....

Connection/Love

....
....

Priorities/Focus/Purpose

....
....
....
....

Date:...............................

Weight:.......................

NUTRITION

Number of Meals............

Protein   YES/NO

Fruit & vegetables   YES/NO

Healthy Fat   YES/NO

Fibre   YES/NO

Apple Cider Vinegar   YES/NO

Supplements   YES/NO

METABOLISM

Cold Exposure   YES/NO

Aerobic Exercise

   ✓   ....
   ✓   ....

Anaerobic Exercise

   ✓   ....
   ✓   ....
   ✓   ....
   ✓   ....
   ✓   ....
   ✓   ....
   ✓   ....

Flexibility Exercise

   ✓   ....
   ✓   ....

TIMING

A Good Night's Sleep YES/NO

Breakfast...........................

Dinner Completed...............

Window...........................

Digital Curfew...................

Bedtime...........................

MINDSET

Relaxation

....
....

Mindful Eating   YES/NO

Gratitude

....
....
....

Self-care & Kindness

....
....

Visualisation   YES/NO

Creativity/Joy/Fun

....
....

Connection/Love

....
....

Priorities/Focus/Purpose

....
....
....
....

Date:.................................

Weight:.......................

NUTRITION

Number of Meals............

Protein	YES/NO
Fruit & vegetables	YES/NO
Healthy Fat	YES/NO
Fibre	YES/NO
Apple Cider Vinegar	YES/NO
Supplements	YES/NO

METABOLISM

Cold Exposure   YES/NO

Aerobic Exercise

✓   ....
✓   ....

Anaerobic Exercise

✓   ....
✓   ....
✓   ....
✓   ....
✓   ....
✓   ....
✓   ....

Flexibility Exercise

✓   ....
✓   ....

WEEKLY REVIEW

Weight:

Review...............................

Weight:

Focus...............................

TIMING:

Review...............................
....
....
....
....

TIMING:

Focus...............................
....
....
....
....

MINDSET:

Review...............................
....
....
....
....
....
....

MINDSET:

Focus...............................
....
....
....
....
....
....

NUTRITION:

Review ....
....
....
....
....
....

NUTRITION:

Focus...............................
....
....
....
....
....

METABOLISM:

Review...............................
....
....
....
....

METABOLISM:

Focus...............................
....
....
....
....

"Beware the barrenness of a busy life."

Socrates

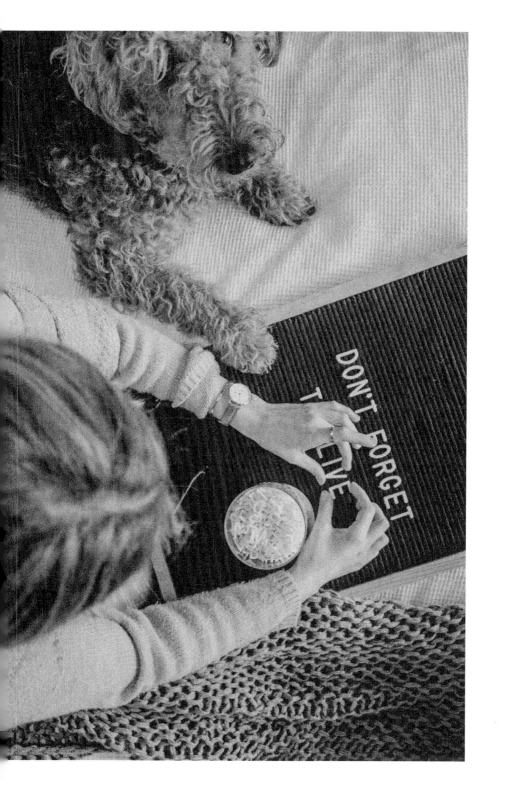

TIMING

A Good Night's Sleep YES/NO

Breakfast...........................

Dinner Completed...............

Window...........................

Digital Curfew...................

Bedtime...........................

MINDSET

Relaxation

....

....

Mindful Eating   YES/NO

Gratitude

....

....

....

Self-care & Kindness

....

....

Visualisation   YES/NO

Creativity/Joy/Fun

....

....

Connection/Love

....

....

Priorities/Focus/Purpose

....

....

....

....

Date:...............................

Weight:.......................

NUTRITION

Number of Meals.............

Protein	YES/NO
Fruit & vegetables	YES/NO
Healthy Fat	YES/NO
Fibre	YES/NO
Apple Cider Vinegar	YES/NO
Supplements	YES/NO

METABOLISM

Cold Exposure   YES/NO

Aerobic Exercise

✓   ....

✓   ....

Anaerobic Exercise

✓   ....

✓   ....

✓   ....

✓   ....

✓   ....

✓   ....

✓   ....

Flexibility Exercise

✓   ....

✓   ....

TIMING

A Good Night's Sleep YES/NO

Breakfast............................

Dinner Completed..............

Window............................

Digital Curfew...................

Bedtime...........................

MINDSET

Relaxation

....

....

Mindful Eating   YES/NO

Gratitude

....

....

....

Self-care & Kindness

....

....

Visualisation   YES/NO

Creativity/Joy/Fun

....

....

Connection/Love

....

....

Priorities/Focus/Purpose

....

....

....

....

Date:..............................

Weight:.......................

NUTRITION

Number of Meals............

Protein   YES/NO

Fruit & vegetables   YES/NO

Healthy Fat   YES/NO

Fibre   YES/NO

Apple Cider Vinegar   YES/NO

Supplements   YES/NO

METABOLISM

Cold Exposure   YES/NO

Aerobic Exercise

✓   ....

✓   ....

Anaerobic Exercise

✓   ....

✓   ....

✓   ....

✓   ....

✓   ....

✓   ....

✓   ....

Flexibility Exercise

✓   ....

✓   ....

TIMING

A Good Night's Sleep YES/NO

Breakfast............................

Dinner Completed...............

Window...........................

Digital Curfew...................

Bedtime............................

MINDSET

Relaxation

....
....

Mindful Eating   YES/NO

Gratitude

....
....
....

Self-care & Kindness

....
....

Visualisation   YES/NO

Creativity/Joy/Fun

....
....

Connection/Love

....
....

Priorities/Focus/Purpose

....
....
....
....

Date:..................................

Weight:.......................

NUTRITION

Number of Meals.............

Protein   YES/NO

Fruit & vegetables   YES/NO

Healthy Fat   YES/NO

Fibre   YES/NO

Apple Cider Vinegar   YES/NO

Supplements   YES/NO

METABOLISM

Cold Exposure   YES/NO

Aerobic Exercise

✓   ....
✓   ....

Anaerobic Exercise

✓   ....
✓   ....
✓   ....
✓   ....
✓   ....
✓   ....
✓   ....

Flexibility Exercise

✓   ....
✓   ....

TIMING

A Good Night's Sleep YES/NO

Breakfast...........................

Dinner Completed...............

Window...........................

Digital Curfew...................

Bedtime...........................

MINDSET

Relaxation

....

....

Mindful Eating   YES/NO

Gratitude

....

....

....

Self-care & Kindness

....

....

Visualisation   YES/NO

Creativity/Joy/Fun

....

....

Connection/Love

....

....

Priorities/Focus/Purpose

....

....

....

....

Date:................................

Weight:........................

NUTRITION

Number of Meals............

Protein	YES/NO
Fruit & vegetables	YES/NO
Healthy Fat	YES/NO
Fibre	YES/NO
Apple Cider Vinegar	YES/NO
Supplements	YES/NO

METABOLISM

Cold Exposure   YES/NO

Aerobic Exercise

  ✓ ....

  ✓ ....

Anaerobic Exercise

  ✓ ....

  ✓ ....

  ✓ ....

  ✓ ....

  ✓ ....

  ✓ ....

  ✓ ....

Flexibility Exercise

  ✓ ....

  ✓ ....

TIMING

A Good Night's Sleep YES/NO

Breakfast..........................

Dinner Completed...............

Window...........................

Digital Curfew...................

Bedtime...........................

MINDSET

Relaxation

....

....

Mindful Eating   YES/NO

Gratitude

....

....

....

Self-care & Kindness

....

....

Visualisation   YES/NO

Creativity/Joy/Fun

....

....

Connection/Love

....

....

Priorities/Focus/Purpose

....

....

....

....

Date:.................................

Weight:........................

NUTRITION

Number of Meals............

Protein	YES/NO
Fruit & vegetables	YES/NO
Healthy Fat	YES/NO
Fibre	YES/NO
Apple Cider Vinegar	YES/NO
Supplements	YES/NO

METABOLISM

Cold Exposure   YES/NO

Aerobic Exercise

✓   ....
✓   ....

Anaerobic Exercise

✓   ....
✓   ....
✓   ....
✓   ....
✓   ....
✓   ....
✓   ....

Flexibility Exercise

✓   ....
✓   ....

TIMING

A Good Night's Sleep YES/NO

Breakfast...........................

Dinner Completed...............

Window...........................

Digital Curfew...................

Bedtime...........................

MINDSET

Relaxation
....
....

Mindful Eating   YES/NO

Gratitude
....
....
....

Self-care & Kindness
....
....

Visualisation   YES/NO

Creativity/Joy/Fun
....
....

Connection/Love
....
....

Priorities/Focus/Purpose
....
....
....
....

Date:...............................

Weight:.......................

NUTRITION

Number of Meals............

Protein	YES/NO
Fruit & vegetables	YES/NO
Healthy Fat	YES/NO
Fibre	YES/NO
Apple Cider Vinegar	YES/NO
Supplements	YES/NO

METABOLISM

Cold Exposure   YES/NO

Aerobic Exercise
   ✓   ....
   ✓   ....

Anaerobic Exercise
   ✓   ....
   ✓   ....
   ✓   ....
   ✓   ....
   ✓   ....
   ✓   ....
   ✓   ....

Flexibility Exercise
   ✓   ....
   ✓   ....

TIMING

A Good Night's Sleep YES/NO

Breakfast...........................

Dinner Completed...............

Window...........................

Digital Curfew...................

Bedtime...........................

MINDSET

Relaxation

....
....

Mindful Eating   YES/NO

Gratitude

....
....
....

Self-care & Kindness

....
....

Visualisation   YES/NO

Creativity/Joy/Fun

....
....

Connection/Love

....
....

Priorities/Focus/Purpose

....
....
....
....

Date:...............................

Weight:.......................

NUTRITION

Number of Meals............

Protein	YES/NO
Fruit & vegetables	YES/NO
Healthy Fat	YES/NO
Fibre	YES/NO
Apple Cider Vinegar	YES/NO
Supplements	YES/NO

METABOLISM

Cold Exposure   YES/NO

Aerobic Exercise

✓ ....
✓ ....

Anaerobic Exercise

✓ ....
✓ ....
✓ ....
✓ ....
✓ ....
✓ ....
✓ ....

Flexibility Exercise

✓ ....
✓ ....

WEEKLY REVIEW

Weight:

Review................................

Weight:

Focus................................

TIMING:

Review................................
....
....
....
....

TIMING:

Focus................................
....
....
....
....

MINDSET:

Review................................
....
....
....
....
....
....

MINDSET:

Focus................................
....
....
....
....

NUTRITION:

Review................................
....
....
....
....
....

NUTRITION:

Focus................................
....
....
....
....

METABOLISM:

Review................................
....
....
....
....

METABOLISM:

Focus................................
....
....
....

"Not what we have but what we enjoy constitutes our abundance."

Epicurus

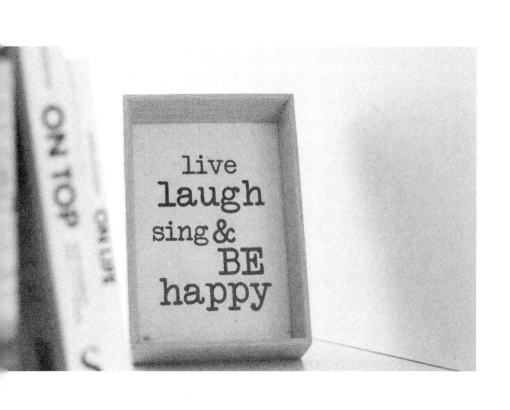

TIMING

A Good Night's Sleep YES/NO

Breakfast............................

Dinner Completed...............

Window...........................

Digital Curfew...................

Bedtime...........................

MINDSET

Relaxation

....
....

Mindful Eating   YES/NO

Gratitude

....
....
....

Self-care & Kindness

....
....

Visualisation   YES/NO

Creativity/Joy/Fun

....
....

Connection/Love

....
....

Priorities/Focus/Purpose

....
....
....
....

Date:...............................

Weight:........................

NUTRITION

Number of Meals.............

Protein	YES/NO
Fruit & vegetables	YES/NO
Healthy Fat	YES/NO
Fibre	YES/NO
Apple Cider Vinegar	YES/NO
Supplements	YES/NO

METABOLISM

Cold Exposure   YES/NO

Aerobic Exercise

✓   ....
✓   ....

Anaerobic Exercise

✓   ....
✓   ....
✓   ....
✓   ....
✓   ....
✓   ....
✓   ....

Flexibility Exercise

✓   ....
✓   ....

TIMING

A Good Night's Sleep YES/NO

Breakfast............................

Dinner Completed...............

Window...........................

Digital Curfew...................

Bedtime............................

MINDSET

Relaxation
....
....

Mindful Eating   YES/NO

Gratitude
....
....
....

Self-care & Kindness
....
....

Visualisation   YES/NO

Creativity/Joy/Fun
....
....

Connection/Love
....
....

Priorities/Focus/Purpose
....
....
....
....

Date:...............................

Weight:........................

NUTRITION

Number of Meals............

Protein	YES/NO
Fruit & vegetables	YES/NO
Healthy Fat	YES/NO
Fibre	YES/NO
Apple Cider Vinegar	YES/NO
Supplements	YES/NO

METABOLISM

Cold Exposure   YES/NO

Aerobic Exercise

✓   ....
✓   ....

Anaerobic Exercise

✓   ....
✓   ....
✓   ....
✓   ....
✓   ....
✓   ....
✓   ....

Flexibility Exercise

✓   ....
✓   ....

TIMING

A Good Night's Sleep YES/NO

Breakfast...........................

Dinner Completed...............

Window...........................

Digital Curfew...................

Bedtime...........................

MINDSET

Relaxation

....

....

Mindful Eating   YES/NO

Gratitude

....

....

....

Self-care & Kindness

....

....

Visualisation   YES/NO

Creativity/Joy/Fun

....

....

Connection/Love

....

....

Priorities/Focus/Purpose

....

....

....

....

Date:................................

Weight:......................

NUTRITION

Number of Meals............

Protein	YES/NO
Fruit & vegetables	YES/NO
Healthy Fat	YES/NO
Fibre	YES/NO
Apple Cider Vinegar	YES/NO
Supplements	YES/NO

METABOLISM

Cold Exposure   YES/NO

Aerobic Exercise

✓   ....

✓   ....

Anaerobic Exercise

✓   ....

✓   ....

✓   ....

✓   ....

✓   ....

✓   ....

✓   ....

Flexibility Exercise

✓   ....

✓   ....

TIMING

A Good Night's Sleep YES/NO

Breakfast...........................

Dinner Completed...............

Window...........................

Digital Curfew...................

Bedtime...........................

MINDSET

Relaxation

....
....

Mindful Eating   YES/NO

Gratitude

....
....
....

Self-care & Kindness

....
....

Visualisation   YES/NO

Creativity/Joy/Fun

....
....

Connection/Love

....
....

Priorities/Focus/Purpose

....
....
....
....

Date:..............................

Weight:......................

NUTRITION

Number of Meals............

Protein	YES/NO
Fruit & vegetables	YES/NO
Healthy Fat	YES/NO
Fibre	YES/NO
Apple Cider Vinegar	YES/NO
Supplements	YES/NO

METABOLISM

Cold Exposure   YES/NO

Aerobic Exercise

✓   ....
✓   ....

Anaerobic Exercise

✓   ....
✓   ....
✓   ....
✓   ....
✓   ....
✓   ....
✓   ....

Flexibility Exercise

✓   ....
✓   ....

TIMING

A Good Night's Sleep YES/NO

Breakfast...........................

Dinner Completed...............

Window............................

Digital Curfew...................

Bedtime...........................

MINDSET

Relaxation
....
....

Mindful Eating   YES/NO

Gratitude
....
....
....

Self-care & Kindness
....
....

Visualisation   YES/NO

Creativity/Joy/Fun
....
....

Connection/Love
....
....

Priorities/Focus/Purpose
....
....
....
....

Date:................................

Weight:........................

NUTRITION

Number of Meals.............

Protein	YES/NO
Fruit & vegetables	YES/NO
Healthy Fat	YES/NO
Fibre	YES/NO
Apple Cider Vinegar	YES/NO
Supplements	YES/NO

METABOLISM

Cold Exposure   YES/NO

Aerobic Exercise
- ✓ ....
- ✓ ....

Anaerobic Exercise
- ✓ ....
- ✓ ....
- ✓ ....
- ✓ ....
- ✓ ....
- ✓ ....
- ✓ ....

Flexibility Exercise
- ✓ ....
- ✓ ....

TIMING

A Good Night's Sleep YES/NO

Breakfast...........................

Dinner Completed...............

Window...........................

Digital Curfew...................

Bedtime............................

MINDSET

Relaxation

....

....

Mindful Eating   YES/NO

Gratitude

....

....

....

Self-care & Kindness

....

....

Visualisation   YES/NO

Creativity/Joy/Fun

....

....

Connection/Love

....

....

Priorities/Focus/Purpose

....

....

....

....

Date:................................

Weight:......................

NUTRITION

Number of Meals............

Protein	YES/NO
Fruit & vegetables	YES/NO
Healthy Fat	YES/NO
Fibre	YES/NO
Apple Cider Vinegar	YES/NO
Supplements	YES/NO

METABOLISM

Cold Exposure   YES/NO

Aerobic Exercise

   ✓   ....

   ✓   ....

Anaerobic Exercise

   ✓   ....

   ✓   ....

   ✓   ....

   ✓   ....

   ✓   ....

   ✓   ....

   ✓   ....

Flexibility Exercise

   ✓   ....

   ✓   ....

TIMING

A Good Night's Sleep YES/NO

Breakfast...........................

Dinner Completed...............

Window...........................

Digital Curfew....................

Bedtime............................

MINDSET

Relaxation

....

....

Mindful Eating   YES/NO

Gratitude

....

....

....

Self-care & Kindness

....

....

Visualisation   YES/NO

Creativity/Joy/Fun

....

....

Connection/Love

....

....

Priorities/Focus/Purpose

....

....

....

....

Date:................................

Weight:.......................

NUTRITION

Number of Meals............

Protein   YES/NO

Fruit & vegetables   YES/NO

Healthy Fat   YES/NO

Fibre   YES/NO

Apple Cider Vinegar   YES/NO

Supplements   YES/NO

METABOLISM

Cold Exposure   YES/NO

Aerobic Exercise

   ✓   ....
   ✓   ....

Anaerobic Exercise

   ✓   ....
   ✓   ....
   ✓   ....
   ✓   ....
   ✓   ....
   ✓   ....
   ✓   ....

Flexibility Exercise

   ✓   ....
   ✓   ....

WEEKLY REVIEW

Weight:	**Weight:**
Review............................	Focus................................

TIMING:	**TIMING:**
Review............................	Focus................................
....	....
....	....
....	....
....	....

MINDSET:	**MINDSET:**
Review............................	Focus................................
....	....
....	....
....	....
....	....
....	....
....	....

NUTRITION:	**NUTRITION:**
Review	Focus................................
....	....
....	....
....	....
....	....
....	....

METABOLISM:	**METABOLISM:**
Review............................	Focus................................
....	....
....	....
....	....

"When you are content to be simply yourself and don't compare or compete, everybody will respect you."

Lao Tzu

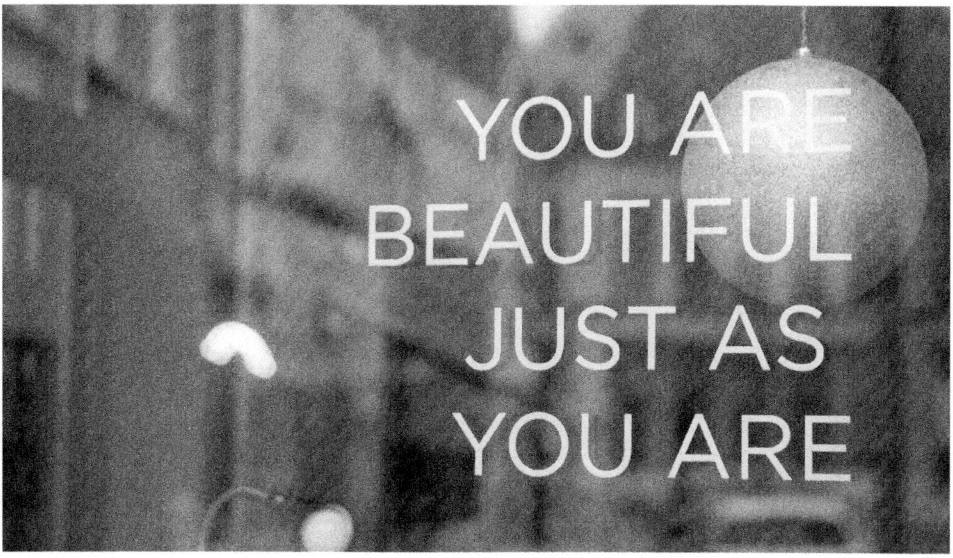
YOU ARE
BEAUTIFUL
JUST AS
YOU ARE

TIMING

A Good Night's Sleep YES/NO

Breakfast...........................

Dinner Completed...............

Window...........................

Digital Curfew...................

Bedtime...........................

MINDSET

Relaxation

....
....

Mindful Eating   YES/NO

Gratitude

....
....
....

Self-care & Kindness

....
....

Visualisation   YES/NO

Creativity/Joy/Fun

....
....

Connection/Love

....
....

Priorities/Focus/Purpose

....
....
....
....

Date:................................

Weight:........................

NUTRITION

Number of Meals............

Protein	YES/NO
Fruit & vegetables	YES/NO
Healthy Fat	YES/NO
Fibre	YES/NO
Apple Cider Vinegar	YES/NO
Supplements	YES/NO

METABOLISM

Cold Exposure   YES/NO

Aerobic Exercise

✓   ....
✓   ....

Anaerobic Exercise

✓   ....
✓   ....
✓   ....
✓   ....
✓   ....
✓   ....
✓   ....

Flexibility Exercise

✓   ....
✓   ....

TIMING

A Good Night's Sleep YES/NO

Breakfast...........................

Dinner Completed...............

Window...........................

Digital Curfew..................

Bedtime...........................

MINDSET

Relaxation
....
....

Mindful Eating   YES/NO

Gratitude
....
....
....

Self-care & Kindness
....
....

Visualisation   YES/NO

Creativity/Joy/Fun
....
....

Connection/Love
....
....

Priorities/Focus/Purpose
....
....
....
....

Date:...............................

Weight:.......................

NUTRITION

Number of Meals............

Protein	YES/NO
Fruit & vegetables	YES/NO
Healthy Fat	YES/NO
Fibre	YES/NO
Apple Cider Vinegar	YES/NO
Supplements	YES/NO

METABOLISM

Cold Exposure   YES/NO

Aerobic Exercise
✓   ....
✓   ....

Anaerobic Exercise
✓   ....
✓   ....
✓   ....
✓   ....
✓   ....
✓   ....
✓   ....

Flexibility Exercise
✓   ....
✓   ....

TIMING

A Good Night's Sleep YES/NO

Breakfast...........................

Dinner Completed...............

Window...........................

Digital Curfew...................

Bedtime...........................

MINDSET

Relaxation

....

....

Mindful Eating   YES/NO

Gratitude

....

....

....

Self-care & Kindness

....

....

Visualisation   YES/NO

Creativity/Joy/Fun

....

....

Connection/Love

....

....

Priorities/Focus/Purpose

....

....

....

....

Date:................................

Weight:......................

NUTRITION

Number of Meals............

Protein	YES/NO
Fruit & vegetables	YES/NO
Healthy Fat	YES/NO
Fibre	YES/NO
Apple Cider Vinegar	YES/NO
Supplements	YES/NO

METABOLISM

Cold Exposure   YES/NO

Aerobic Exercise

   ✓   ....
   ✓   ....

Anaerobic Exercise

   ✓   ....
   ✓   ....
   ✓   ....
   ✓   ....
   ✓   ....
   ✓   ....
   ✓   ....

Flexibility Exercise

   ✓   ....
   ✓   ....

TIMING

A Good Night's Sleep YES/NO

Breakfast...........................

Dinner Completed...............

Window...........................

Digital Curfew...................

Bedtime...........................

MINDSET

Relaxation
....
....

Mindful Eating   YES/NO

Gratitude
....
....
....

Self-care & Kindness
....
....

Visualisation   YES/NO

Creativity/Joy/Fun
....
....

Connection/Love
....
....

Priorities/Focus/Purpose
....
....
....
....

Date:...............................

Weight:.......................

NUTRITION

Number of Meals............	
Protein	YES/NO
Fruit & vegetables	YES/NO
Healthy Fat	YES/NO
Fibre	YES/NO
Apple Cider Vinegar	YES/NO
Supplements	YES/NO

METABOLISM

Cold Exposure   YES/NO

Aerobic Exercise
- ✓ ....
- ✓ ....

Anaerobic Exercise
- ✓ ....
- ✓ ....
- ✓ ....
- ✓ ....
- ✓ ....
- ✓ ....
- ✓ ....

Flexibility Exercise
- ✓ ....
- ✓ ....

TIMING

A Good Night's Sleep YES/NO

Breakfast...........................

Dinner Completed...............

Window...........................

Digital Curfew...................

Bedtime...........................

MINDSET

Relaxation

....

....

Mindful Eating   YES/NO

Gratitude

....

....

....

Self-care & Kindness

....

....

Visualisation   YES/NO

Creativity/Joy/Fun

....

....

Connection/Love

....

....

Priorities/Focus/Purpose

....

....

....

....

Date:...............................

Weight:.......................

NUTRITION

Number of Meals............

Protein	YES/NO
Fruit & vegetables	YES/NO
Healthy Fat	YES/NO
Fibre	YES/NO
Apple Cider Vinegar	YES/NO
Supplements	YES/NO

METABOLISM

Cold Exposure   YES/NO

Aerobic Exercise

   ✓ ....

   ✓ ....

Anaerobic Exercise

   ✓ ....

   ✓ ....

   ✓ ....

   ✓ ....

   ✓ ....

   ✓ ....

   ✓ ....

Flexibility Exercise

   ✓ ....

   ✓ ....

TIMING

A Good Night's Sleep YES/NO

Breakfast..........................

Dinner Completed...............

Window...........................

Digital Curfew...................

Bedtime...........................

MINDSET

Relaxation
....
....

Mindful Eating   YES/NO

Gratitude
....
....
....

Self-care & Kindness
....
....

Visualisation   YES/NO

Creativity/Joy/Fun
....
....

Connection/Love
....
....

Priorities/Focus/Purpose
....
....
....
....

Date:..................................

Weight:......................

NUTRITION

Number of Meals............

Protein	YES/NO
Fruit & vegetables	YES/NO
Healthy Fat	YES/NO
Fibre	YES/NO
Apple Cider Vinegar	YES/NO
Supplements	YES/NO

METABOLISM

Cold Exposure   YES/NO

Aerobic Exercise
 ✓ ....
 ✓ ....

Anaerobic Exercise
 ✓ ....
 ✓ ....
 ✓ ....
 ✓ ....
 ✓ ....
 ✓ ....
 ✓ ....

Flexibility Exercise
 ✓ ....
 ✓ ....

TIMING

A Good Night's Sleep YES/NO

Breakfast..............................

Dinner Completed...............

Window............................

Digital Curfew....................

Bedtime...........................

MINDSET

Relaxation

....
....

Mindful Eating   YES/NO

Gratitude

....
....
....

Self-care & Kindness

....
....

Visualisation   YES/NO

Creativity/Joy/Fun

....
....

Connection/Love

....
....

Priorities/Focus/Purpose

....
....
....
....

Date:...............................

Weight:.......................

NUTRITION

Number of Meals.............

Protein	YES/NO
Fruit & vegetables	YES/NO
Healthy Fat	YES/NO
Fibre	YES/NO
Apple Cider Vinegar	YES/NO
Supplements	YES/NO

METABOLISM

Cold Exposure   YES/NO

Aerobic Exercise

✓   ....
✓   ....

Anaerobic Exercise

✓   ....
✓   ....
✓   ....
✓   ....
✓   ....
✓   ....
✓   ....

Flexibility Exercise

✓   ....
✓   ....

WEEKLY REVIEW

Weight:

Review.................................

Weight:

Focus.................................

TIMING:

Review.................................
....
....
....
....

TIMING:

Focus.................................
....
....
....
....

MINDSET:

Review.................................
....
....
....
....
....
....

MINDSET:

Focus.................................
....
....
....
....
....

NUTRITION:

Review ....
....
....
....
....
....

NUTRITION:

Focus.................................
....
....
....
....

METABOLISM:

Review.................................
....
....
....
....

METABOLISM:

Focus.................................
....
....
....

"Everything that happens happens as it should, and if you observe carefully, you will find this to be so."

Marcus Aurelius

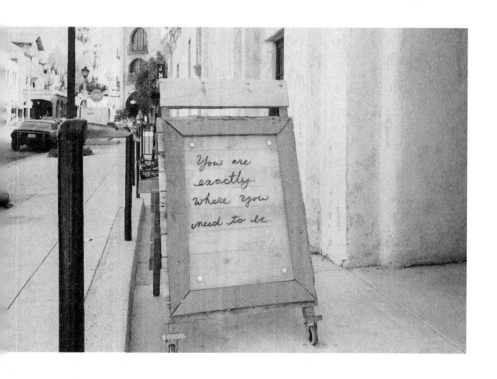

TIMING

A Good Night's Sleep YES/NO

Breakfast...........................

Dinner Completed...............

Window...........................

Digital Curfew...................

Bedtime...........................

MINDSET

Relaxation

....
....

Mindful Eating   YES/NO

Gratitude

....
....
....

Self-care & Kindness

....
....

Visualisation   YES/NO

Creativity/Joy/Fun

....
....

Connection/Love

....
....

Priorities/Focus/Purpose

....
....
....
....

Date:...............................

Weight:......................

NUTRITION

Number of Meals............

Protein   YES/NO

Fruit & vegetables   YES/NO

Healthy Fat   YES/NO

Fibre   YES/NO

Apple Cider Vinegar   YES/NO

Supplements   YES/NO

METABOLISM

Cold Exposure   YES/NO

Aerobic Exercise

✓   ....
✓   ....

Anaerobic Exercise

✓   ....
✓   ....
✓   ....
✓   ....
✓   ....
✓   ....
✓   ....

Flexibility Exercise

✓   ....
✓   ....

TIMING

A Good Night's Sleep YES/NO

Breakfast...........................

Dinner Completed...............

Window...........................

Digital Curfew...................

Bedtime...........................

MINDSET

Relaxation
....
....

Mindful Eating   YES/NO

Gratitude
....
....
....

Self-care & Kindness
....
....

Visualisation   YES/NO

Creativity/Joy/Fun
....
....

Connection/Love
....
....

Priorities/Focus/Purpose
....
....
....
....

Date:...............................

Weight:......................

NUTRITION

Number of Meals............

Protein	YES/NO
Fruit & vegetables	YES/NO
Healthy Fat	YES/NO
Fibre	YES/NO
Apple Cider Vinegar	YES/NO
Supplements	YES/NO

METABOLISM

Cold Exposure   YES/NO

Aerobic Exercise
   ✓ ....
   ✓ ....

Anaerobic Exercise
   ✓ ....
   ✓ ....
   ✓ ....
   ✓ ....
   ✓ ....
   ✓ ....
   ✓ ....

Flexibility Exercise
   ✓ ....
   ✓ ....

TIMING

A Good Night's Sleep YES/NO

Breakfast...........................

Dinner Completed...............

Window...........................

Digital Curfew...................

Bedtime...........................

MINDSET

Relaxation

....
....

Mindful Eating   YES/NO

Gratitude

....
....
....

Self-care & Kindness

....
....

Visualisation   YES/NO

Creativity/Joy/Fun

....
....

Connection/Love

....
....

Priorities/Focus/Purpose

....
....
....
....

Date:..............................

Weight:.......................

NUTRITION

Number of Meals.............

Protein	YES/NO
Fruit & vegetables	YES/NO
Healthy Fat	YES/NO
Fibre	YES/NO
Apple Cider Vinegar	YES/NO
Supplements	YES/NO

METABOLISM

Cold Exposure   YES/NO

Aerobic Exercise

✓ ....
✓ ....

Anaerobic Exercise

✓ ....
✓ ....
✓ ....
✓ ....
✓ ....
✓ ....
✓ ....

Flexibility Exercise

✓ ....
✓ ....

TIMING

A Good Night's Sleep YES/NO

Breakfast...........................

Dinner Completed...............

Window............................

Digital Curfew...................

Bedtime............................

MINDSET

Relaxation
....
....

Mindful Eating   YES/NO

Gratitude
....
....
....

Self-care & Kindness
....
....

Visualisation   YES/NO

Creativity/Joy/Fun
....
....

Connection/Love
....
....

Priorities/Focus/Purpose
....
....
....
....

Date:...............................

Weight:.......................

NUTRITION

Number of Meals............

Protein	YES/NO
Fruit & vegetables	YES/NO
Healthy Fat	YES/NO
Fibre	YES/NO
Apple Cider Vinegar	YES/NO
Supplements	YES/NO

METABOLISM

Cold Exposure   YES/NO

Aerobic Exercise
✓   ....
✓   ....

Anaerobic Exercise
✓   ....
✓   ....
✓   ....
✓   ....
✓   ....
✓   ....
✓   ....

Flexibility Exercise
✓   ....
✓   ....

TIMING

A Good Night's Sleep YES/NO

Breakfast...........................

Dinner Completed..............

Window..........................

Digital Curfew...................

Bedtime..........................

MINDSET

Relaxation

....

....

Mindful Eating   YES/NO

Gratitude

....

....

....

Self-care & Kindness

....

....

Visualisation   YES/NO

Creativity/Joy/Fun

....

....

Connection/Love

....

....

Priorities/Focus/Purpose

....

....

....

....

Date:...............................

Weight:.....................

NUTRITION

Number of Meals............

Protein	YES/NO
Fruit & vegetables	YES/NO
Healthy Fat	YES/NO
Fibre	YES/NO
Apple Cider Vinegar	YES/NO
Supplements	YES/NO

METABOLISM

Cold Exposure   YES/NO

Aerobic Exercise

✓   ....

✓   ....

Anaerobic Exercise

✓   ....

✓   ....

✓   ....

✓   ....

✓   ....

✓   ....

✓   ....

Flexibility Exercise

✓   ....

✓   ....

TIMING

A Good Night's Sleep YES/NO

Breakfast.............................

Dinner Completed...............

Window............................

Digital Curfew...................

Bedtime............................

MINDSET

Relaxation

....

....

Mindful Eating   YES/NO

Gratitude

....

....

....

Self-care & Kindness

....

....

Visualisation   YES/NO

Creativity/Joy/Fun

....

....

Connection/Love

....

....

Priorities/Focus/Purpose

....

....

....

....

Date:...............................

Weight:........................

NUTRITION

Number of Meals............

Protein	YES/NO
Fruit & vegetables	YES/NO
Healthy Fat	YES/NO
Fibre	YES/NO
Apple Cider Vinegar	YES/NO
Supplements	YES/NO

METABOLISM

Cold Exposure   YES/NO

Aerobic Exercise

✓   ....
✓   ....

Anaerobic Exercise

✓   ....
✓   ....
✓   ....
✓   ....
✓   ....
✓   ....
✓   ....

Flexibility Exercise

✓   ....
✓   ....

TIMING

A Good Night's Sleep YES/NO

Breakfast...........................

Dinner Completed................

Window..............................

Digital Curfew....................

Bedtime.............................

MINDSET

Relaxation

....
....

Mindful Eating   YES/NO

Gratitude

....
....
....

Self-care & Kindness

....
....

Visualisation   YES/NO

Creativity/Joy/Fun

....
....

Connection/Love

....
....

Priorities/Focus/Purpose

....
....
....
....

Date:...................................

Weight:.......................

NUTRITION

Number of Meals............

Protein	YES/NO
Fruit & vegetables	YES/NO
Healthy Fat	YES/NO
Fibre	YES/NO
Apple Cider Vinegar	YES/NO
Supplements	YES/NO

METABOLISM

Cold Exposure   YES/NO

Aerobic Exercise

✓ ....
✓ ....

Anaerobic Exercise

✓ ....
✓ ....
✓ ....
✓ ....
✓ ....
✓ ....
✓ ....

Flexibility Exercise

✓ ....
✓ ....

WEEKLY REVIEW

Weight:	**Weight:**
Review.............................	Focus.............................

TIMING:	**TIMING:**
Review............................	Focus............................
....	....
....	....
....	....
....	....

MINDSET:	**MINDSET:**
Review............................	Focus............................
....	....
....	....
....	....
....	....
....	....
....	....

NUTRITION:	**NUTRITION:**
Review	Focus............................
....	....
....	....
....	....
....	....
....	....

METABOLISM:	**METABOLISM:**
Review............................	Focus............................
....	....
....	....
....	....
....	....

"I've heard there are troubles of more than one kind; some come from ahead, and some come from behind. But I've brought a big bat. I'm all ready, you see; now my troubles are going to have troubles with me!"

Dr. Seuss

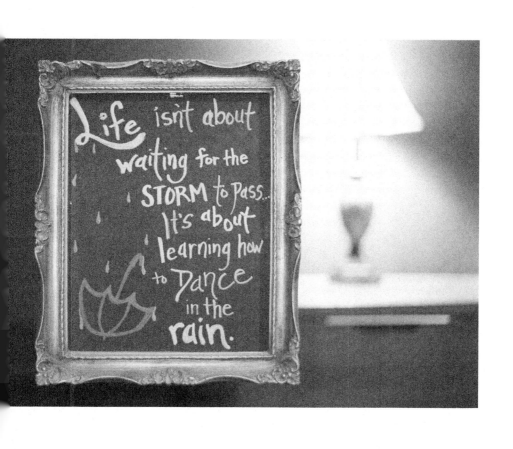

TIMING

A Good Night's Sleep YES/NO

Breakfast...........................

Dinner Completed...............

Window...........................

Digital Curfew....................

Bedtime...........................

Date:.................................

Weight:.......................

NUTRITION

Number of Meals............

Protein	YES/NO
Fruit & vegetables	YES/NO
Healthy Fat	YES/NO
Fibre	YES/NO
Apple Cider Vinegar	YES/NO
Supplements	YES/NO

MINDSET

Relaxation
....
....

Mindful Eating   YES/NO

Gratitude
....
....
....

Self-care & Kindness
....
....

Visualisation   YES/NO

Creativity/Joy/Fun
....
....

Connection/Love
....
....

Priorities/Focus/Purpose
....
....
....
....

METABOLISM

Cold Exposure   YES/NO

Aerobic Exercise
  ✓ ....
  ✓ ....

Anaerobic Exercise
  ✓ ....
  ✓ ....
  ✓ ....
  ✓ ....
  ✓ ....
  ✓ ....
  ✓ ....

Flexibility Exercise
  ✓ ....
  ✓ ....

TIMING

A Good Night's Sleep YES/NO

Breakfast.............................

Dinner Completed...............

Window...........................

Digital Curfew...................

Bedtime...........................

MINDSET

Relaxation
....
....

Mindful Eating   YES/NO

Gratitude
....
....
....

Self-care & Kindness
....
....

Visualisation   YES/NO

Creativity/Joy/Fun
....
....

Connection/Love
....
....

Priorities/Focus/Purpose
....
....
....
....

Date:...............................

Weight:.......................

NUTRITION

Number of Meals............

Protein	YES/NO
Fruit & vegetables	YES/NO
Healthy Fat	YES/NO
Fibre	YES/NO
Apple Cider Vinegar	YES/NO
Supplements	YES/NO

METABOLISM

Cold Exposure   YES/NO

Aerobic Exercise
   ✓ ....
   ✓ ....

Anaerobic Exercise
   ✓ ....
   ✓ ....
   ✓ ....
   ✓ ....
   ✓ ....
   ✓ ....
   ✓ ....

Flexibility Exercise
   ✓ ....
   ✓ ....

TIMING

A Good Night's Sleep YES/NO

Breakfast...........................

Dinner Completed...............

Window...........................

Digital Curfew...................

Bedtime...........................

MINDSET

Relaxation
....
....

Mindful Eating   YES/NO

Gratitude
....
....
....

Self-care & Kindness
....
....

Visualisation   YES/NO

Creativity/Joy/Fun
....
....

Connection/Love
....
....

Priorities/Focus/Purpose
....
....
....
....

Date:.............................

Weight:......................

NUTRITION

Number of Meals............

Protein	YES/NO
Fruit & vegetables	YES/NO
Healthy Fat	YES/NO
Fibre	YES/NO
Apple Cider Vinegar	YES/NO
Supplements	YES/NO

METABOLISM

Cold Exposure   YES/NO

Aerobic Exercise
   ✓ ....
   ✓ ....

Anaerobic Exercise
   ✓ ....
   ✓ ....
   ✓ ....
   ✓ ....
   ✓ ....
   ✓ ....
   ✓ ....

Flexibility Exercise
   ✓ ....
   ✓ ....

TIMING

A Good Night's Sleep YES/NO

Breakfast...........................

Dinner Completed...............

Window...........................

Digital Curfew...................

Bedtime...........................

MINDSET

Relaxation
....
....

Mindful Eating   YES/NO

Gratitude
....
....
....

Self-care & Kindness
....
....

Visualisation   YES/NO

Creativity/Joy/Fun
....
....

Connection/Love
....
....

Priorities/Focus/Purpose
....
....
....
....

Date:.................................

Weight:......................

NUTRITION

Number of Meals............

Protein	YES/NO
Fruit & vegetables	YES/NO
Healthy Fat	YES/NO
Fibre	YES/NO
Apple Cider Vinegar	YES/NO
Supplements	YES/NO

METABOLISM

Cold Exposure   YES/NO

Aerobic Exercise
✓   ....
✓   ....

Anaerobic Exercise
✓   ....
✓   ....
✓   ....
✓   ....
✓   ....
✓   ....
✓   ....

Flexibility Exercise
✓   ....
✓   ....

TIMING

A Good Night's Sleep YES/NO

Breakfast..........................

Dinner Completed...............

Window...........................

Digital Curfew...................

Bedtime...........................

Date:.................................

Weight:.......................

NUTRITION

Number of Meals.............

Protein	YES/NO
Fruit & vegetables	YES/NO
Healthy Fat	YES/NO
Fibre	YES/NO
Apple Cider Vinegar	YES/NO
Supplements	YES/NO

MINDSET

Relaxation
....
....

Mindful Eating   YES/NO

Gratitude
....
....
....

Self-care & Kindness
....
....

Visualisation   YES/NO

Creativity/Joy/Fun
....
....

Connection/Love
....
....

Priorities/Focus/Purpose
....
....
....
....

METABOLISM

Cold Exposure   YES/NO

Aerobic Exercise
✓ ....
✓ ....

Anaerobic Exercise
✓ ....
✓ ....
✓ ....
✓ ....
✓ ....
✓ ....
✓ ....

Flexibility Exercise
✓ ....
✓ ....

TIMING

A Good Night's Sleep YES/NO

Breakfast...........................

Dinner Completed...............

Window...........................

Digital Curfew...................

Bedtime...........................

MINDSET

Relaxation
....
....

Mindful Eating   YES/NO

Gratitude
....
....
....

Self-care & Kindness
....
....

Visualisation   YES/NO

Creativity/Joy/Fun
....
....

Connection/Love
....
....

Priorities/Focus/Purpose
....
....
....
....

Date:................................

Weight:.......................

NUTRITION

Number of Meals............

Protein	YES/NO
Fruit & vegetables	YES/NO
Healthy Fat	YES/NO
Fibre	YES/NO
Apple Cider Vinegar	YES/NO
Supplements	YES/NO

METABOLISM

Cold Exposure   YES/NO

Aerobic Exercise
   ✓ ....
   ✓ ....

Anaerobic Exercise
   ✓ ....
   ✓ ....
   ✓ ....
   ✓ ....
   ✓ ....
   ✓ ....
   ✓ ....

Flexibility Exercise
   ✓ ....
   ✓ ....

TIMING

A Good Night's Sleep YES/NO

Breakfast...........................

Dinner Completed...............

Window...........................

Digital Curfew...................

Bedtime...........................

MINDSET

Relaxation

....

....

Mindful Eating   YES/NO

Gratitude

....

....

....

Self-care & Kindness

....

....

Visualisation   YES/NO

Creativity/Joy/Fun

....

....

Connection/Love

....

....

Priorities/Focus/Purpose

....

....

....

....

Date:...............................

Weight:.......................

NUTRITION

Number of Meals............

Protein	YES/NO
Fruit & vegetables	YES/NO
Healthy Fat	YES/NO
Fibre	YES/NO
Apple Cider Vinegar	YES/NO
Supplements	YES/NO

METABOLISM

Cold Exposure   YES/NO

Aerobic Exercise

✓   ....
✓   ....

Anaerobic Exercise

✓   ....
✓   ....
✓   ....
✓   ....
✓   ....
✓   ....
✓   ....

Flexibility Exercise

✓   ....
✓   ....

WEEKLY REVIEW

Weight:	**Weight:**
Review...............................	Focus...............................

TIMING:	**TIMING:**
Review...............................	Focus...............................
....	....
....	....
....	....
....	....

MINDSET:	**MINDSET:**
Review...............................	Focus...............................
....	....
....	....
....	....
....	....
....	....
....	....

NUTRITION:	**NUTRITION:**
Review	Focus...............................
....	....
....	....
....	....
....	....

METABOLISM:	**METABOLISM:**
Review...............................	Focus...............................
....	....
....	....
....	....
....	....

"Our greatest glory is not in never falling, but in rising every time we fall."

Confucius

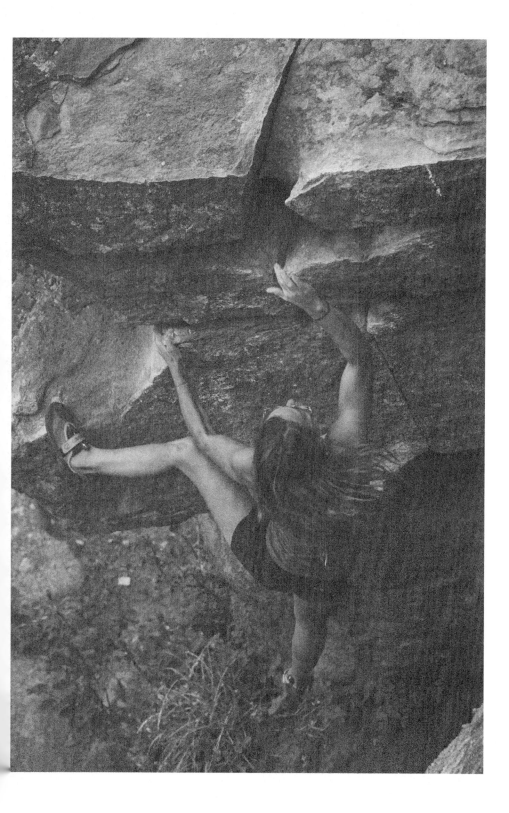

TIMING

A Good Night's Sleep YES/NO

Breakfast............................

Dinner Completed...............

Window.............................

Digital Curfew....................

Bedtime............................

Date:...............................

Weight:.........................

NUTRITION

Number of Meals.............

Protein	YES/NO
Fruit & vegetables	YES/NO
Healthy Fat	YES/NO
Fibre	YES/NO
Apple Cider Vinegar	YES/NO
Supplements	YES/NO

MINDSET

Relaxation

....
....

Mindful Eating   YES/NO

Gratitude

....
....
....

Self-care & Kindness

....
....

Visualisation   YES/NO

Creativity/Joy/Fun

....
....

Connection/Love

....
....

Priorities/Focus/Purpose

....
....
....
....

METABOLISM

Cold Exposure   YES/NO

Aerobic Exercise

✓   ....
✓   ....

Anaerobic Exercise

✓   ....
✓   ....
✓   ....
✓   ....
✓   ....
✓   ....
✓   ....

Flexibility Exercise

✓   ....
✓   ....

TIMING

A Good Night's Sleep YES/NO

Breakfast...........................

Dinner Completed...............

Window............................

Digital Curfew...................

Bedtime...........................

MINDSET

Relaxation
....
....

Mindful Eating   YES/NO

Gratitude
....
....
....

Self-care & Kindness
....
....

Visualisation   YES/NO

Creativity/Joy/Fun
....
....

Connection/Love
....
....

Priorities/Focus/Purpose
....
....
....
....

Date:...............................

Weight:.......................

NUTRITION

Number of Meals............

Protein	YES/NO
Fruit & vegetables	YES/NO
Healthy Fat	YES/NO
Fibre	YES/NO
Apple Cider Vinegar	YES/NO
Supplements	YES/NO

METABOLISM

Cold Exposure   YES/NO

Aerobic Exercise

✓ ....
✓ ....

Anaerobic Exercise

✓ ....
✓ ....
✓ ....
✓ ....
✓ ....
✓ ....
✓ ....

Flexibility Exercise

✓ ....
✓ ....

TIMING

A Good Night's Sleep YES/NO

Breakfast...........................

Dinner Completed...............

Window...........................

Digital Curfew...................

Bedtime...........................

MINDSET

Relaxation
....
....

Mindful Eating   YES/NO

Gratitude
....
....
....

Self-care & Kindness
....
....

Visualisation   YES/NO

Creativity/Joy/Fun
....
....

Connection/Love
....
....

Priorities/Focus/Purpose
....
....
....
....

Date:................................

Weight:.......................

NUTRITION

Number of Meals............

Protein   YES/NO

Fruit & vegetables   YES/NO

Healthy Fat   YES/NO

Fibre   YES/NO

Apple Cider Vinegar   YES/NO

Supplements   YES/NO

METABOLISM

Cold Exposure   YES/NO

Aerobic Exercise
   ✓ ....
   ✓ ....

Anaerobic Exercise
   ✓ ....
   ✓ ....
   ✓ ....
   ✓ ....
   ✓ ....
   ✓ ....
   ✓ ....

Flexibility Exercise
   ✓ ....
   ✓ ....

TIMING

A Good Night's Sleep YES/NO

Breakfast.............................

Dinner Completed...............

Window............................

Digital Curfew....................

Bedtime............................

MINDSET

Relaxation

....

....

Mindful Eating   YES/NO

Gratitude

....

....

....

Self-care & Kindness

....

....

Visualisation   YES/NO

Creativity/Joy/Fun

....

....

Connection/Love

....

....

Priorities/Focus/Purpose

....

....

....

....

Date:...............................

Weight:........................

NUTRITION

Number of Meals............

Protein	YES/NO
Fruit & vegetables	YES/NO
Healthy Fat	YES/NO
Fibre	YES/NO
Apple Cider Vinegar	YES/NO
Supplements	YES/NO

METABOLISM

Cold Exposure   YES/NO

Aerobic Exercise

✓   ....

✓   ....

Anaerobic Exercise

✓   ....

✓   ....

✓   ....

✓   ....

✓   ....

✓   ....

✓   ....

Flexibility Exercise

✓   ....

✓   ....

TIMING

A Good Night's Sleep YES/NO

Breakfast..........................

Dinner Completed...............

Window...........................

Digital Curfew...................

Bedtime..........................

MINDSET

Relaxation
....
....

Mindful Eating   YES/NO

Gratitude
....
....
....

Self-care & Kindness
....
....

Visualisation   YES/NO

Creativity/Joy/Fun
....
....

Connection/Love
....
....

Priorities/Focus/Purpose
....
....
....
....

Date:...............................

Weight:......................

NUTRITION

Number of Meals............

Protein   YES/NO

Fruit & vegetables   YES/NO

Healthy Fat   YES/NO

Fibre   YES/NO

Apple Cider Vinegar   YES/NO

Supplements   YES/NO

METABOLISM

Cold Exposure   YES/NO

Aerobic Exercise
✓   ....
✓   ....

Anaerobic Exercise
✓   ....
✓   ....
✓   ....
✓   ....
✓   ....
✓   ....
✓   ....

Flexibility Exercise
✓   ....
✓   ....

TIMING

A Good Night's Sleep YES/NO

Breakfast............................

Dinner Completed...............

Window............................

Digital Curfew...................

Bedtime............................

MINDSET

Relaxation

....

....

Mindful Eating   YES/NO

Gratitude

....

....

....

Self-care & Kindness

....

....

Visualisation   YES/NO

Creativity/Joy/Fun

....

....

Connection/Love

....

....

Priorities/Focus/Purpose

....

....

....

....

Date:................................

Weight:.....................

NUTRITION

Number of Meals............

Protein	YES/NO
Fruit & vegetables	YES/NO
Healthy Fat	YES/NO
Fibre	YES/NO
Apple Cider Vinegar	YES/NO
Supplements	YES/NO

METABOLISM

Cold Exposure   YES/NO

Aerobic Exercise

✓ ....
✓ ....

Anaerobic Exercise

✓ ....
✓ ....
✓ ....
✓ ....
✓ ....
✓ ....
✓ ....

Flexibility Exercise

✓ ....
✓ ....

TIMING

A Good Night's Sleep YES/NO

Breakfast...........................

Dinner Completed...............

Window............................

Digital Curfew...................

Bedtime...........................

MINDSET

Relaxation
....
....

Mindful Eating   YES/NO

Gratitude
....
....
....

Self-care & Kindness
....
....

Visualisation   YES/NO

Creativity/Joy/Fun
....
....

Connection/Love
....
....

Priorities/Focus/Purpose
....
....
....
....

Date:................................

Weight:........................

NUTRITION

Number of Meals............

Protein   YES/NO

Fruit & vegetables   YES/NO

Healthy Fat   YES/NO

Fibre   YES/NO

Apple Cider Vinegar   YES/NO

Supplements   YES/NO

METABOLISM

Cold Exposure   YES/NO

Aerobic Exercise
   ✓   ....
   ✓   ....

Anaerobic Exercise
   ✓   ....
   ✓   ....
   ✓   ....
   ✓   ....
   ✓   ....
   ✓   ....
   ✓   ....

Flexibility Exercise
   ✓   ....
   ✓   ....

WEEKLY REVIEW

Weight:

Review...........................

Weight:

Focus................................

TIMING:

Review...............................
....
....
....
....

TIMING:

Focus...............................
....
....
....
....

MINDSET:

Review...............................
....
....
....
....
....
....

MINDSET:

Focus...............................
....
....
....
....
....
....

NUTRITION:

Review ....
....
....
....
....
....

NUTRITION:

Focus...............................
....
....
....
....

METABOLISM:

Review...............................
....
....
....
....

METABOLISM:

Focus...............................
....
....
....
....

"It may be hard for an egg to turn into a bird: it would be a jolly sight harder for it to learn to fly while remaining an egg."

C. S. Lewis

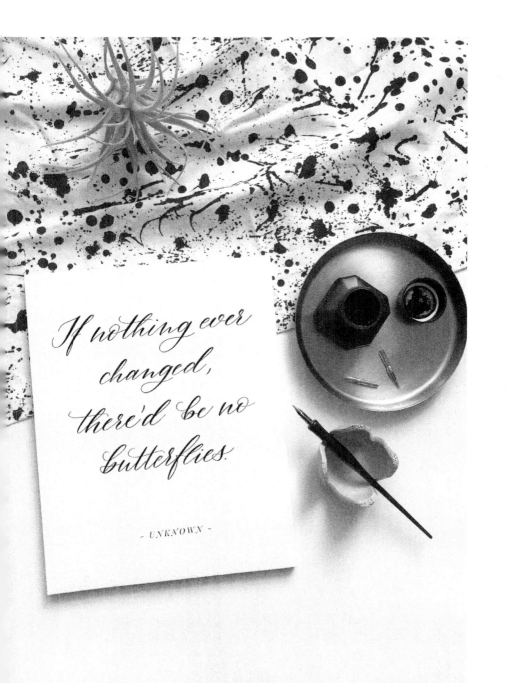

TIMING

A Good Night's Sleep YES/NO

Breakfast...........................

Dinner Completed...............

Window...........................

Digital Curfew....................

Bedtime...........................

MINDSET

Relaxation

....

....

Mindful Eating   YES/NO

Gratitude

....

....

....

Self-care & Kindness

....

....

Visualisation   YES/NO

Creativity/Joy/Fun

....

....

Connection/Love

....

....

Priorities/Focus/Purpose

....

....

....

....

Date:................................

Weight:........................

NUTRITION

Number of Meals............

Protein	YES/NO
Fruit & vegetables	YES/NO
Healthy Fat	YES/NO
Fibre	YES/NO
Apple Cider Vinegar	YES/NO
Supplements	YES/NO

METABOLISM

Cold Exposure   YES/NO

Aerobic Exercise

✓   ....

✓   ....

Anaerobic Exercise

✓   ....

✓   ....

✓   ....

✓   ....

✓   ....

✓   ....

✓   ....

Flexibility Exercise

✓   ....

✓   ....

TIMING

A Good Night's Sleep YES/NO

Breakfast...........................

Dinner Completed...............

Window............................

Digital Curfew....................

Bedtime............................

MINDSET

Relaxation

....
....

Mindful Eating   YES/NO

Gratitude

....
....
....

Self-care & Kindness

....
....

Visualisation   YES/NO

Creativity/Joy/Fun

....
....

Connection/Love

....
....

Priorities/Focus/Purpose

....
....
....
....

Date:...............................

Weight:.......................

NUTRITION

Number of Meals............

Protein	YES/NO
Fruit & vegetables	YES/NO
Healthy Fat	YES/NO
Fibre	YES/NO
Apple Cider Vinegar	YES/NO
Supplements	YES/NO

METABOLISM

Cold Exposure   YES/NO

Aerobic Exercise

✓   ....
✓   ....

Anaerobic Exercise

✓   ....
✓   ....
✓   ....
✓   ....
✓   ....
✓   ....
✓   ....

Flexibility Exercise

✓   ....
✓   ....

TIMING

A Good Night's Sleep YES/NO

Breakfast...........................

Dinner Completed................

Window............................

Digital Curfew....................

Bedtime............................

MINDSET

Relaxation

....

....

Mindful Eating   YES/NO

Gratitude

....

....

....

Self-care & Kindness

....

....

Visualisation   YES/NO

Creativity/Joy/Fun

....

....

Connection/Love

....

....

Priorities/Focus/Purpose

....

....

....

....

Date:...............................

Weight:.......................

NUTRITION

Number of Meals.............

Protein	YES/NO
Fruit & vegetables	YES/NO
Healthy Fat	YES/NO
Fibre	YES/NO
Apple Cider Vinegar	YES/NO
Supplements	YES/NO

METABOLISM

Cold Exposure   YES/NO

Aerobic Exercise

✓ ....

✓ ....

Anaerobic Exercise

✓ ....

✓ ....

✓ ....

✓ ....

✓ ....

✓ ....

✓ ....

Flexibility Exercise

✓ ....

✓ ....

TIMING

A Good Night's Sleep YES/NO

Breakfast...........................

Dinner Completed..............

Window...........................

Digital Curfew...................

Bedtime...........................

MINDSET

Relaxation
....
....

Mindful Eating   YES/NO

Gratitude
....
....
....

Self-care & Kindness
....
....

Visualisation   YES/NO

Creativity/Joy/Fun
....
....

Connection/Love
....
....

Priorities/Focus/Purpose
....
....
....
....

Date:................................

Weight:.......................

NUTRITION

Number of Meals............

Protein	YES/NO
Fruit & vegetables	YES/NO
Healthy Fat	YES/NO
Fibre	YES/NO
Apple Cider Vinegar	YES/NO
Supplements	YES/NO

METABOLISM

Cold Exposure   YES/NO

Aerobic Exercise
    ✓ ....
    ✓ ....

Anaerobic Exercise
    ✓ ....
    ✓ ....
    ✓ ....
    ✓ ....
    ✓ ....
    ✓ ....
    ✓ ....

Flexibility Exercise
    ✓ ....
    ✓ ....

TIMING

A Good Night's Sleep YES/NO

Breakfast...........................

Dinner Completed...............

Window...........................

Digital Curfew...................

Bedtime...........................

MINDSET

Relaxation

....

....

Mindful Eating   YES/NO

Gratitude

....

....

....

Self-care & Kindness

....

....

Visualisation   YES/NO

Creativity/Joy/Fun

....

....

Connection/Love

....

....

Priorities/Focus/Purpose

....

....

....

....

Date:...............................

Weight:.......................

NUTRITION

Number of Meals............

Protein	YES/NO
Fruit & vegetables	YES/NO
Healthy Fat	YES/NO
Fibre	YES/NO
Apple Cider Vinegar	YES/NO
Supplements	YES/NO

METABOLISM

Cold Exposure   YES/NO

Aerobic Exercise

✓ ....

✓ ....

Anaerobic Exercise

✓ ....

✓ ....

✓ ....

✓ ....

✓ ....

✓ ....

✓ ....

Flexibility Exercise

✓ ....

✓ ....

TIMING

A Good Night's Sleep YES/NO

Breakfast...........................

Dinner Completed...............

Window...........................

Digital Curfew...................

Bedtime...........................

MINDSET

Relaxation
....
....

Mindful Eating   YES/NO

Gratitude
....
....
....

Self-care & Kindness
....
....

Visualisation   YES/NO

Creativity/Joy/Fun
....
....

Connection/Love
....
....

Priorities/Focus/Purpose
....
....
....
....

Date:...............................

Weight:.......................

NUTRITION

Number of Meals............

Protein	YES/NO
Fruit & vegetables	YES/NO
Healthy Fat	YES/NO
Fibre	YES/NO
Apple Cider Vinegar	YES/NO
Supplements	YES/NO

METABOLISM

Cold Exposure   YES/NO

Aerobic Exercise
   ✓ ....
   ✓ ....

Anaerobic Exercise
   ✓ ....
   ✓ ....
   ✓ ....
   ✓ ....
   ✓ ....
   ✓ ....
   ✓ ....

Flexibility Exercise
   ✓ ....
   ✓ ....

TIMING

A Good Night's Sleep YES/NO

Breakfast...........................

Dinner Completed...............

Window...........................

Digital Curfew...................

Bedtime...........................

MINDSET

Relaxation

....
....

Mindful Eating   YES/NO

Gratitude

....
....
....

Self-care & Kindness

....
....

Visualisation   YES/NO

Creativity/Joy/Fun

....
....

Connection/Love

....
....

Priorities/Focus/Purpose

....
....
....
....

Date:...............................

Weight:.......................

NUTRITION

Number of Meals.............

Protein   YES/NO

Fruit & vegetables   YES/NO

Healthy Fat   YES/NO

Fibre   YES/NO

Apple Cider Vinegar   YES/NO

Supplements   YES/NO

METABOLISM

Cold Exposure   YES/NO

Aerobic Exercise

   ✓   ....
   ✓   ....

Anaerobic Exercise

   ✓   ....
   ✓   ....
   ✓   ....
   ✓   ....
   ✓   ....
   ✓   ....
   ✓   ....

Flexibility Exercise

   ✓   ....
   ✓   ....

WEEKLY REVIEW

Weight:

Review...............................

Weight:

Focus...............................

TIMING:

Review................................
....
....
....
....

TIMING:

Focus................................
....
....
....
....

MINDSET:

Review................................
....
....
....
....
....
....

MINDSET:

Focus................................
....
....
....
....
....
....

NUTRITION:

Review ....
....
....
....
....
....

NUTRITION:

Focus................................
....
....
....
....
....

METABOLISM:

Review................................
....
....
....
....

METABOLISM:

Focus................................
....
....
....
....

"When I let go of what I am,
I become what I might be."

Lao Tzu

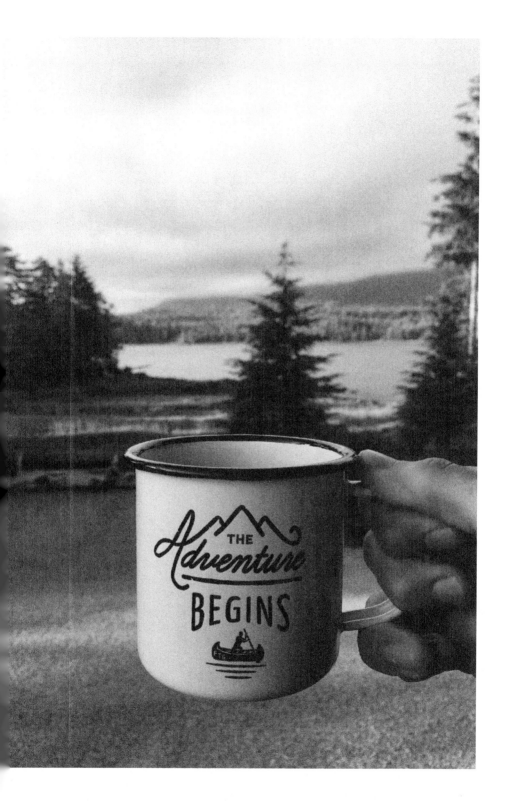

TIMING

A Good Night's Sleep YES/NO

Breakfast...........................

Dinner Completed...............

Window...........................

Digital Curfew....................

Bedtime............................

MINDSET

Relaxation

....

....

Mindful Eating   YES/NO

Gratitude

....

....

....

Self-care & Kindness

....

....

Visualisation   YES/NO

Creativity/Joy/Fun

....

....

Connection/Love

....

....

Priorities/Focus/Purpose

....

....

....

....

Date:................................

Weight:......................

NUTRITION

Number of Meals............

Protein	YES/NO
Fruit & vegetables	YES/NO
Healthy Fat	YES/NO
Fibre	YES/NO
Apple Cider Vinegar	YES/NO
Supplements	YES/NO

METABOLISM

Cold Exposure   YES/NO

Aerobic Exercise

✓ ....

✓ ....

Anaerobic Exercise

✓ ....

✓ ....

✓ ....

✓ ....

✓ ....

✓ ....

✓ ....

Flexibility Exercise

✓ ....

✓ ....

TIMING

A Good Night's Sleep YES/NO

Breakfast...........................

Dinner Completed...............

Window...........................

Digital Curfew...................

Bedtime...........................

MINDSET

Relaxation
....
....

Mindful Eating   YES/NO

Gratitude
....
....
....

Self-care & Kindness
....
....

Visualisation   YES/NO

Creativity/Joy/Fun
....
....

Connection/Love
....
....

Priorities/Focus/Purpose
....
....
....
....

Date:...............................

Weight:.......................

NUTRITION

Number of Meals............

Protein	YES/NO
Fruit & vegetables	YES/NO
Healthy Fat	YES/NO
Fibre	YES/NO
Apple Cider Vinegar	YES/NO
Supplements	YES/NO

METABOLISM

Cold Exposure   YES/NO

Aerobic Exercise
✓   ....
✓   ....

Anaerobic Exercise
✓   ....
✓   ....
✓   ....
✓   ....
✓   ....
✓   ....
✓   ....

Flexibility Exercise
✓   ....
✓   ....

TIMING

A Good Night's Sleep YES/NO

Breakfast...........................

Dinner Completed...............

Window...........................

Digital Curfew...................

Bedtime...........................

MINDSET

Relaxation

....
....

Mindful Eating   YES/NO

Gratitude

....
....
....

Self-care & Kindness

....
....

Visualisation   YES/NO

Creativity/Joy/Fun

....
....

Connection/Love

....
....

Priorities/Focus/Purpose

....
....
....
....

Date:..................................

Weight:.......................

NUTRITION

Number of Meals............

Protein   YES/NO

Fruit & vegetables   YES/NO

Healthy Fat   YES/NO

Fibre   YES/NO

Apple Cider Vinegar   YES/NO

Supplements   YES/NO

METABOLISM

Cold Exposure   YES/NO

Aerobic Exercise

✓ ....
✓ ....

Anaerobic Exercise

✓ ....
✓ ....
✓ ....
✓ ....
✓ ....
✓ ....
✓ ....

Flexibility Exercise

✓ ....
✓ ....

TIMING

A Good Night's Sleep YES/NO

Breakfast...........................

Dinner Completed..............

Window...........................

Digital Curfew...................

Bedtime...........................

MINDSET

Relaxation
....
....

Mindful Eating   YES/NO

Gratitude
....
....
....

Self-care & Kindness
....
....

Visualisation   YES/NO

Creativity/Joy/Fun
....
....

Connection/Love
....
....

Priorities/Focus/Purpose
....
....
....
....

Date:...............................

Weight:......................

NUTRITION

Number of Meals............

Protein	YES/NO
Fruit & vegetables	YES/NO
Healthy Fat	YES/NO
Fibre	YES/NO
Apple Cider Vinegar	YES/NO
Supplements	YES/NO

METABOLISM

Cold Exposure   YES/NO

Aerobic Exercise

✓   ....
✓   ....

Anaerobic Exercise

✓   ....
✓   ....
✓   ....
✓   ....
✓   ....
✓   ....
✓   ....

Flexibility Exercise

✓   ....
✓   ....

TIMING

A Good Night's Sleep YES/NO

Breakfast...........................

Dinner Completed...............

Window...........................

Digital Curfew...................

Bedtime...........................

MINDSET

Relaxation
....
....

Mindful Eating   YES/NO

Gratitude
....
....
....

Self-care & Kindness
....
....

Visualisation   YES/NO

Creativity/Joy/Fun
....
....

Connection/Love
....
....

Priorities/Focus/Purpose
....
....
....
....

Date:................................

Weight:........................

NUTRITION

Number of Meals............

Protein   YES/NO

Fruit & vegetables   YES/NO

Healthy Fat   YES/NO

Fibre   YES/NO

Apple Cider Vinegar   YES/NO

Supplements   YES/NO

METABOLISM

Cold Exposure   YES/NO

Aerobic Exercise
  ✓   ....
  ✓   ....

Anaerobic Exercise
  ✓   ....
  ✓   ....
  ✓   ....
  ✓   ....
  ✓   ....
  ✓   ....
  ✓   ....

Flexibility Exercise
  ✓   ....
  ✓   ....

TIMING

A Good Night's Sleep YES/NO

Breakfast...........................

Dinner Completed...............

Window...........................

Digital Curfew..................

Bedtime............................

MINDSET

Relaxation

....

....

Mindful Eating   YES/NO

Gratitude

....

....

....

Self-care & Kindness

....

....

Visualisation   YES/NO

Creativity/Joy/Fun

....

....

Connection/Love

....

....

Priorities/Focus/Purpose

....

....

....

....

Date:.................................

Weight:.......................

NUTRITION

Number of Meals............

Protein	YES/NO
Fruit & vegetables	YES/NO
Healthy Fat	YES/NO
Fibre	YES/NO
Apple Cider Vinegar	YES/NO
Supplements	YES/NO

METABOLISM

Cold Exposure   YES/NO

Aerobic Exercise

✓   ....

✓   ....

Anaerobic Exercise

✓   ....

✓   ....

✓   ....

✓   ....

✓   ....

✓   ....

✓   ....

Flexibility Exercise

✓   ....

✓   ....

TIMING

A Good Night's Sleep YES/NO

Breakfast...........................

Dinner Completed...............

Window..........................

Digital Curfew...................

Bedtime...........................

MINDSET

Relaxation

....

....

Mindful Eating   YES/NO

Gratitude

....

....

....

Self-care & Kindness

....

....

Visualisation   YES/NO

Creativity/Joy/Fun

....

....

Connection/Love

....

....

Priorities/Focus/Purpose

....

....

....

....

Date:................................

Weight:.....................

NUTRITION

Number of Meals............

Protein   YES/NO

Fruit & vegetables   YES/NO

Healthy Fat   YES/NO

Fibre   YES/NO

Apple Cider Vinegar   YES/NO

Supplements   YES/NO

METABOLISM

Cold Exposure   YES/NO

Aerobic Exercise

✓   ....

✓   ....

Anaerobic Exercise

✓   ....

✓   ....

✓   ....

✓   ....

✓   ....

✓   ....

✓   ....

Flexibility Exercise

✓   ....

✓   ....

WEEKLY REVIEW

Weight:

Review..............................

Weight:

Focus..............................

TIMING:

Review..............................
....
....
....
....

TIMING:

Focus..............................
....
....
....
....

MINDSET:

Review..............................
....
....
....
....
....
....

MINDSET:

Focus..............................
....
....
....
....
....
....

NUTRITION:

Review ....
....
....
....
....
....

NUTRITION:

Focus..............................
....
....
....
....

METABOLISM:

Review..............................
....
....
....
....

METABOLISM:

Focus..............................
....
....
....
....

"It is one of the beautiful compensations in this life that no one can sincerely try to help another without helping himself."

Ralph Waldo Emerson

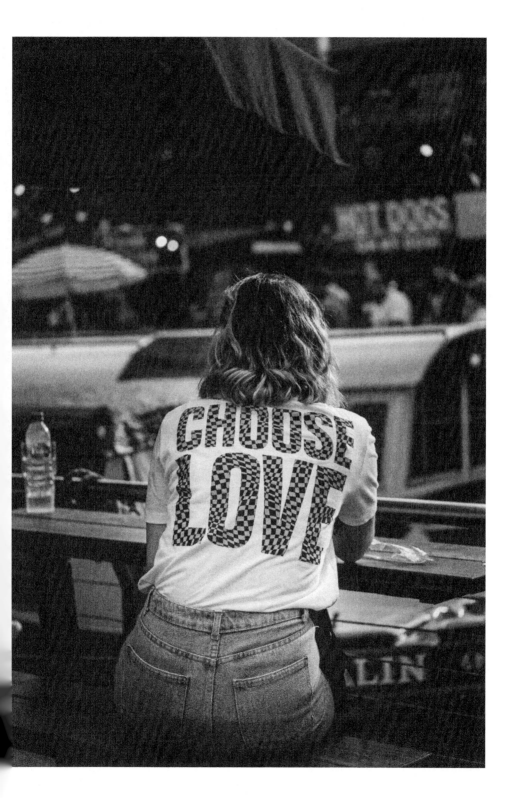

TIMING

A Good Night's Sleep YES/NO

Breakfast............................

Dinner Completed...............

Window...........................

Digital Curfew...................

Bedtime...........................

MINDSET

Relaxation

....

....

Mindful Eating   YES/NO

Gratitude

....

....

....

Self-care & Kindness

....

....

Visualisation   YES/NO

Creativity/Joy/Fun

....

....

Connection/Love

....

....

Priorities/Focus/Purpose

....

....

....

....

Date:...............................

Weight:.......................

NUTRITION

Number of Meals............

Protein   YES/NO

Fruit & vegetables   YES/NO

Healthy Fat   YES/NO

Fibre   YES/NO

Apple Cider Vinegar   YES/NO

Supplements   YES/NO

METABOLISM

Cold Exposure   YES/NO

Aerobic Exercise

✓   ....

✓   ....

Anaerobic Exercise

✓   ....

✓   ....

✓   ....

✓   ....

✓   ....

✓   ....

✓   ....

Flexibility Exercise

✓   ....

✓   ....

TIMING

A Good Night's Sleep YES/NO

Breakfast...........................

Dinner Completed...............

Window...........................

Digital Curfew...................

Bedtime............................

MINDSET

Relaxation

....
....

Mindful Eating   YES/NO

Gratitude

....
....
....

Self-care & Kindness

....
....

Visualisation   YES/NO

Creativity/Joy/Fun

....
....

Connection/Love

....
....

Priorities/Focus/Purpose

....
....
....
....

Date:...................................

Weight:........................

NUTRITION

Number of Meals............

Protein	YES/NO
Fruit & vegetables	YES/NO
Healthy Fat	YES/NO
Fibre	YES/NO
Apple Cider Vinegar	YES/NO
Supplements	YES/NO

METABOLISM

Cold Exposure   YES/NO

Aerobic Exercise

✓   ....
✓   ....

Anaerobic Exercise

✓   ....
✓   ....
✓   ....
✓   ....
✓   ....
✓   ....
✓   ....

Flexibility Exercise

✓   ....
✓   ....

TIMING

A Good Night's Sleep YES/NO

Breakfast...........................

Dinner Completed..............

Window..........................

Digital Curfew...................

Bedtime..........................

MINDSET

Relaxation

....
....

Mindful Eating   YES/NO

Gratitude

....
....
....

Self-care & Kindness

....
....

Visualisation   YES/NO

Creativity/Joy/Fun

....
....

Connection/Love

....
....

Priorities/Focus/Purpose

....
....
....
....

Date:...............................

Weight:......................

NUTRITION

Number of Meals............

Protein	YES/NO
Fruit & vegetables	YES/NO
Healthy Fat	YES/NO
Fibre	YES/NO
Apple Cider Vinegar	YES/NO
Supplements	YES/NO

METABOLISM

Cold Exposure   YES/NO

Aerobic Exercise

✓   ....
✓   ....

Anaerobic Exercise

✓   ....
✓   ....
✓   ....
✓   ....
✓   ....
✓   ....
✓   ....

Flexibility Exercise

✓   ....
✓   ....

TIMING

A Good Night's Sleep YES/NO

Breakfast...........................

Dinner Completed..............

Window...........................

Digital Curfew...................

Bedtime...........................

MINDSET

Relaxation
....
....

Mindful Eating   YES/NO

Gratitude
....
....
....

Self-care & Kindness
....
....

Visualisation   YES/NO

Creativity/Joy/Fun
....
....

Connection/Love
....
....

Priorities/Focus/Purpose
....
....
....
....

Date:...............................

Weight:......................

NUTRITION

Number of Meals............

Protein	YES/NO
Fruit & vegetables	YES/NO
Healthy Fat	YES/NO
Fibre	YES/NO
Apple Cider Vinegar	YES/NO
Supplements	YES/NO

METABOLISM

Cold Exposure   YES/NO

Aerobic Exercise
  ✓ ....
  ✓ ....

Anaerobic Exercise
  ✓ ....
  ✓ ....
  ✓ ....
  ✓ ....
  ✓ ....
  ✓ ....
  ✓ ....

Flexibility Exercise
  ✓ ....
  ✓ ....

TIMING

A Good Night's Sleep YES/NO

Breakfast...........................

Dinner Completed...............

Window...........................

Digital Curfew...................

Bedtime...........................

MINDSET

Relaxation

....

....

Mindful Eating   YES/NO

Gratitude

....

....

....

Self-care & Kindness

....

....

Visualisation   YES/NO

Creativity/Joy/Fun

....

....

Connection/Love

....

....

Priorities/Focus/Purpose

....

....

....

....

Date:...............................

Weight:.......................

NUTRITION

Number of Meals............

Protein	YES/NO
Fruit & vegetables	YES/NO
Healthy Fat	YES/NO
Fibre	YES/NO
Apple Cider Vinegar	YES/NO
Supplements	YES/NO

METABOLISM

Cold Exposure   YES/NO

Aerobic Exercise

   ✓ ....

   ✓ ....

Anaerobic Exercise

   ✓ ....

   ✓ ....

   ✓ ....

   ✓ ....

   ✓ ....

   ✓ ....

   ✓ ....

Flexibility Exercise

   ✓ ....

   ✓ ....

TIMING

A Good Night's Sleep YES/NO

Breakfast...........................

Dinner Completed...............

Window...........................

Digital Curfew...................

Bedtime...........................

MINDSET

Relaxation
....
....

Mindful Eating   YES/NO

Gratitude
....
....
....

Self-care & Kindness
....
....

Visualisation   YES/NO

Creativity/Joy/Fun
....
....

Connection/Love
....
....

Priorities/Focus/Purpose
....
....
....
....

Date:...............................

Weight:......................

NUTRITION

Number of Meals............

Protein	YES/NO
Fruit & vegetables	YES/NO
Healthy Fat	YES/NO
Fibre	YES/NO
Apple Cider Vinegar	YES/NO
Supplements	YES/NO

METABOLISM

Cold Exposure   YES/NO

Aerobic Exercise
- ✓ ....
- ✓ ....

Anaerobic Exercise
- ✓ ....
- ✓ ....
- ✓ ....
- ✓ ....
- ✓ ....
- ✓ ....
- ✓ ....

Flexibility Exercise
- ✓ ....
- ✓ ....

TIMING

A Good Night's Sleep YES/NO

Breakfast...........................

Dinner Completed...............

Window...........................

Digital Curfew...................

Bedtime...........................

MINDSET

Relaxation
....
....

Mindful Eating   YES/NO

Gratitude
....
....
....

Self-care & Kindness
....
....

Visualisation   YES/NO

Creativity/Joy/Fun
....
....

Connection/Love
....
....

Priorities/Focus/Purpose
....
....
....
....

Date:...............................

Weight:.......................

NUTRITION

Number of Meals............

Protein   YES/NO

Fruit & vegetables   YES/NO

Healthy Fat   YES/NO

Fibre   YES/NO

Apple Cider Vinegar   YES/NO

Supplements   YES/NO

METABOLISM

Cold Exposure   YES/NO

Aerobic Exercise
   ✓   ....
   ✓   ....

Anaerobic Exercise
   ✓   ....
   ✓   ....
   ✓   ....
   ✓   ....
   ✓   ....
   ✓   ....
   ✓   ....

Flexibility Exercise
   ✓   ....
   ✓   ....

WEEKLY REVIEW

Weight:

Review.............................

Weight:

Focus..............................

TIMING:

Review.............................
....
....
....
....

TIMING:

Focus..............................
....
....
....
....

MINDSET:

Review.............................
....
....
....
....
....
....

MINDSET:

Focus..............................
....
....
....
....
....
....

NUTRITION:

Review ....
....
....
....
....
....

NUTRITION:

Focus..............................
....
....
....
....
....

METABOLISM:

Review.............................
....
....
....
....

METABOLISM:

Focus..............................
....
....
....
....

"Thought and theory must precede all salutary action; yet action is nobler in itself than either thought or theory."

Virginia Woolf

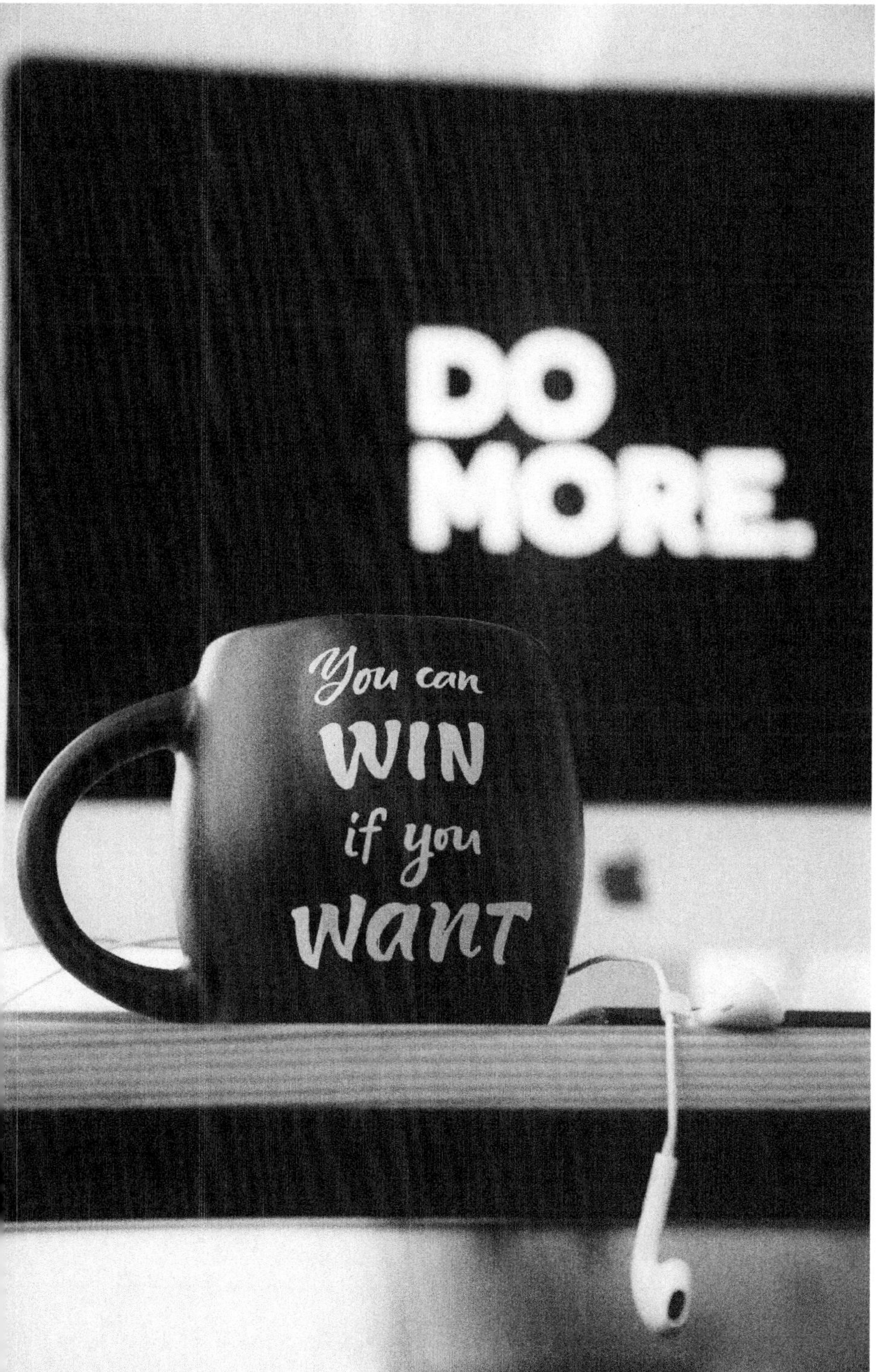
DO
MORE.
You can
WIN
if you
WANT

TIMING

A Good Night's Sleep YES/NO

Breakfast...........................

Dinner Completed...............

Window...........................

Digital Curfew...................

Bedtime...........................

MINDSET

Relaxation

....
....

Mindful Eating   YES/NO

Gratitude

....
....
....

Self-care & Kindness

....
....

Visualisation   YES/NO

Creativity/Joy/Fun

....
....

Connection/Love

....
....

Priorities/Focus/Purpose

....
....
....
....

Date:.............................

Weight:.......................

NUTRITION

Number of Meals............

Protein	YES/NO
Fruit & vegetables	YES/NO
Healthy Fat	YES/NO
Fibre	YES/NO
Apple Cider Vinegar	YES/NO
Supplements	YES/NO

METABOLISM

Cold Exposure   YES/NO

Aerobic Exercise

✓   ....
✓   ....

Anaerobic Exercise

✓   ....
✓   ....
✓   ....
✓   ....
✓   ....
✓   ....
✓   ....

Flexibility Exercise

✓   ....
✓   ....

TIMING

A Good Night's Sleep YES/NO

Breakfast............................

Dinner Completed...............

Window...........................

Digital Curfew....................

Bedtime...........................

MINDSET

Relaxation

....

....

Mindful Eating   YES/NO

Gratitude

....

....

....

Self-care & Kindness

....

....

Visualisation   YES/NO

Creativity/Joy/Fun

....

....

Connection/Love

....

....

Priorities/Focus/Purpose

....

....

....

....

Date:.................................

Weight:.......................

NUTRITION

Number of Meals.............

Protein	YES/NO
Fruit & vegetables	YES/NO
Healthy Fat	YES/NO
Fibre	YES/NO
Apple Cider Vinegar	YES/NO
Supplements	YES/NO

METABOLISM

Cold Exposure   YES/NO

Aerobic Exercise

✓ ....
✓ ....

Anaerobic Exercise

✓ ....
✓ ....
✓ ....
✓ ....
✓ ....
✓ ....
✓ ....

Flexibility Exercise

✓ ....
✓ ....

TIMING

A Good Night's Sleep YES/NO

Breakfast.........................

Dinner Completed...............

Window...........................

Digital Curfew...................

Bedtime...........................

MINDSET

Relaxation

....

....

Mindful Eating   YES/NO

Gratitude

....

....

....

Self-care & Kindness

....

....

Visualisation   YES/NO

Creativity/Joy/Fun

....

....

Connection/Love

....

....

Priorities/Focus/Purpose

....

....

....

....

Date:...............................

Weight:.......................

NUTRITION

Number of Meals............

Protein   YES/NO

Fruit & vegetables   YES/NO

Healthy Fat   YES/NO

Fibre   YES/NO

Apple Cider Vinegar   YES/NO

Supplements   YES/NO

METABOLISM

Cold Exposure   YES/NO

Aerobic Exercise

✓ ....

✓ ....

Anaerobic Exercise

✓ ....

✓ ....

✓ ....

✓ ....

✓ ....

✓ ....

✓ ....

Flexibility Exercise

✓ ....

✓ ....

TIMING

A Good Night's Sleep YES/NO

Breakfast...........................

Dinner Completed...............

Window...........................

Digital Curfew...................

Bedtime...........................

MINDSET

Relaxation
....
....

Mindful Eating   YES/NO

Gratitude
....
....
....

Self-care & Kindness
....
....

Visualisation   YES/NO

Creativity/Joy/Fun
....
....

Connection/Love
....
....

Priorities/Focus/Purpose
....
....
....
....

Date:...............................

Weight:.......................

NUTRITION

Number of Meals............

Protein	YES/NO
Fruit & vegetables	YES/NO
Healthy Fat	YES/NO
Fibre	YES/NO
Apple Cider Vinegar	YES/NO
Supplements	YES/NO

METABOLISM

Cold Exposure   YES/NO

Aerobic Exercise
   ✓ ....
   ✓ ....

Anaerobic Exercise
   ✓ ....
   ✓ ....
   ✓ ....
   ✓ ....
   ✓ ....
   ✓ ....
   ✓ ....

Flexibility Exercise
   ✓ ....
   ✓ ....

TIMING

A Good Night's Sleep YES/NO

Breakfast…………………………

Dinner Completed……………

Window………………………

Digital Curfew…………………

Bedtime………………………

MINDSET

Relaxation

…………………………………

…………………………………

Mindful Eating   YES/NO

Gratitude

…………………………………

…………………………………

…………………………………

Self-care & Kindness

…………………………………

…………………………………

Visualisation   YES/NO

Creativity/Joy/Fun

…………………………………

…………………………………

Connection/Love

…………………………………

…………………………………

Priorities/Focus/Purpose

…………………………………

…………………………………

…………………………………

…………………………………

Date:………………………….

Weight:………………………..

NUTRITION

Number of Meals…………

Protein	YES/NO
Fruit & vegetables	YES/NO
Healthy Fat	YES/NO
Fibre	YES/NO
Apple Cider Vinegar	YES/NO
Supplements	YES/NO

METABOLISM

Cold Exposure   YES/NO

Aerobic Exercise

✓ …………………………

✓ …………………………

Anaerobic Exercise

✓ …………………………

✓ …………………………

✓ …………………………

✓ …………………………

✓ …………………………

✓ …………………………

✓ …………………………

Flexibility Exercise

✓ …………………………

✓ …………………………

TIMING

A Good Night's Sleep YES/NO

Breakfast............................

Dinner Completed...............

Window...........................

Digital Curfew...................

Bedtime............................

MINDSET

Relaxation
....
....

Mindful Eating   YES/NO

Gratitude
....
....
....

Self-care & Kindness
....
....

Visualisation   YES/NO

Creativity/Joy/Fun
....
....

Connection/Love
....
....

Priorities/Focus/Purpose
....
....
....
....

Date:................................

Weight:........................

NUTRITION

Number of Meals............

Protein	YES/NO
Fruit & vegetables	YES/NO
Healthy Fat	YES/NO
Fibre	YES/NO
Apple Cider Vinegar	YES/NO
Supplements	YES/NO

METABOLISM

Cold Exposure   YES/NO

Aerobic Exercise
   ✓   ....
   ✓   ....

Anaerobic Exercise
   ✓   ....
   ✓   ....
   ✓   ....
   ✓   ....
   ✓   ....
   ✓   ....
   ✓   ....

Flexibility Exercise
   ✓   ....
   ✓   ....

TIMING

A Good Night's Sleep YES/NO

Breakfast...........................

Dinner Completed...............

Window...........................

Digital Curfew...................

Bedtime...........................

MINDSET

Relaxation

....
....

Mindful Eating   YES/NO

Gratitude

....
....
....

Self-care & Kindness

....
....

Visualisation   YES/NO

Creativity/Joy/Fun

....
....

Connection/Love

....
....

Priorities/Focus/Purpose

....
....
....
....

Date:.................................

Weight:.......................

NUTRITION

Number of Meals............

Protein	YES/NO
Fruit & vegetables	YES/NO
Healthy Fat	YES/NO
Fibre	YES/NO
Apple Cider Vinegar	YES/NO
Supplements	YES/NO

METABOLISM

Cold Exposure   YES/NO

Aerobic Exercise

✓   ....
✓   ....

Anaerobic Exercise

✓   ....
✓   ....
✓   ....
✓   ....
✓   ....
✓   ....
✓   ....

Flexibility Exercise

✓   ....
✓   ....

WEEKLY REVIEW

Weight:

Review.................................

Weight:

Focus.................................

TIMING:

Review.................................
....
....
....
....

TIMING:

Focus.................................
....
....
....
....

MINDSET:

Review.................................
....
....
....
....
....
....

MINDSET:

Focus.................................
....
....
....
....
....
....

NUTRITION:

Review.................................
....
....
....
....
....

NUTRITION:

Focus.................................
....
....
....
....
....

METABOLISM:

Review.................................
....
....
....
....

METABOLISM:

Focus.................................
....
....
....
....

"Avoiding danger is no safer in the long run than outright exposure. The fearful are caught as often as the bold."

Helen Keller

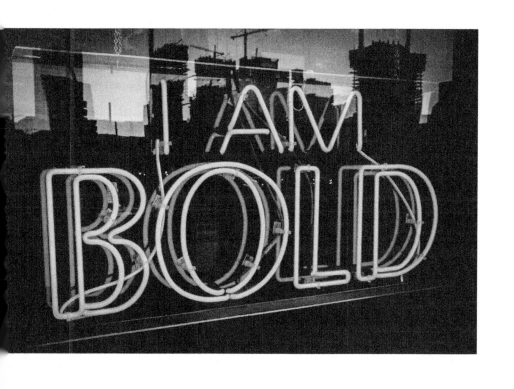

TIMING

A Good Night's Sleep YES/NO

Breakfast...........................

Dinner Completed...............

Window...........................

Digital Curfew...................

Bedtime...........................

MINDSET

Relaxation
....
....

Mindful Eating   YES/NO

Gratitude
....
....
....

Self-care & Kindness
....
....

Visualisation   YES/NO

Creativity/Joy/Fun
....
....

Connection/Love
....
....

Priorities/Focus/Purpose
....
....
....
....

Date:................................

Weight:........................

NUTRITION

Number of Meals............

Protein	YES/NO
Fruit & vegetables	YES/NO
Healthy Fat	YES/NO
Fibre	YES/NO
Apple Cider Vinegar	YES/NO
Supplements	YES/NO

METABOLISM

Cold Exposure   YES/NO

Aerobic Exercise
- ✓ ....
- ✓ ....

Anaerobic Exercise
- ✓ ....
- ✓ ....
- ✓ ....
- ✓ ....
- ✓ ....
- ✓ ....
- ✓ ....

Flexibility Exercise
- ✓ ....
- ✓ ....

TIMING

A Good Night's Sleep YES/NO

Breakfast...........................

Dinner Completed...............

Window...........................

Digital Curfew...................

Bedtime...........................

MINDSET

Relaxation
....
....

Mindful Eating   YES/NO

Gratitude
....
....
....

Self-care & Kindness
....
....

Visualisation   YES/NO

Creativity/Joy/Fun
....
....

Connection/Love
....
....

Priorities/Focus/Purpose
....
....
....
....

Date:...............................

Weight:.......................

NUTRITION

Number of Meals............

Protein	YES/NO
Fruit & vegetables	YES/NO
Healthy Fat	YES/NO
Fibre	YES/NO
Apple Cider Vinegar	YES/NO
Supplements	YES/NO

METABOLISM

Cold Exposure   YES/NO

Aerobic Exercise

✓   ....
✓   ....

Anaerobic Exercise

✓   ....
✓   ....
✓   ....
✓   ....
✓   ....
✓   ....
✓   ....

Flexibility Exercise

✓   ....
✓   ....

TIMING

A Good Night's Sleep YES/NO

Breakfast...........................

Dinner Completed...............

Window...........................

Digital Curfew...................

Bedtime...........................

MINDSET

Relaxation
....
....

Mindful Eating   YES/NO

Gratitude
....
....
....

Self-care & Kindness
....
....

Visualisation   YES/NO

Creativity/Joy/Fun
....
....

Connection/Love
....
....

Priorities/Focus/Purpose
....
....
....
....

Date:...............................

Weight:......................

NUTRITION

Number of Meals............

Protein   YES/NO

Fruit & vegetables   YES/NO

Healthy Fat   YES/NO

Fibre   YES/NO

Apple Cider Vinegar   YES/NO

Supplements   YES/NO

METABOLISM

Cold Exposure   YES/NO

Aerobic Exercise
 ✓ ....
 ✓ ....

Anaerobic Exercise
 ✓ ....
 ✓ ....
 ✓ ....
 ✓ ....
 ✓ ....
 ✓ ....
 ✓ ....

Flexibility Exercise
 ✓ ....
 ✓ ....

TIMING

A Good Night's Sleep YES/NO

Breakfast...........................

Dinner Completed..............

Window..........................

Digital Curfew...................

Bedtime...........................

MINDSET

Relaxation
....
....

Mindful Eating   YES/NO

Gratitude
....
....
....

Self-care & Kindness
....
....

Visualisation   YES/NO

Creativity/Joy/Fun
....
....

Connection/Love
....
....

Priorities/Focus/Purpose
....
....
....
....

Date:...............................

Weight:........................

NUTRITION

Number of Meals............

Protein	YES/NO
Fruit & vegetables	YES/NO
Healthy Fat	YES/NO
Fibre	YES/NO
Apple Cider Vinegar	YES/NO
Supplements	YES/NO

METABOLISM

Cold Exposure   YES/NO

Aerobic Exercise
✓   ....
✓   ....

Anaerobic Exercise
✓   ....
✓   ....
✓   ....
✓   ....
✓   ....
✓   ....
✓   ....

Flexibility Exercise
✓   ....
✓   ....

TIMING

A Good Night's Sleep YES/NO

Breakfast…………………………

Dinner Completed……………

Window………………………

Digital Curfew………………

Bedtime………………………

MINDSET

Relaxation

…………………………………

…………………………………

Mindful Eating   YES/NO

Gratitude

…………………………………

…………………………………

…………………………………

Self-care & Kindness

…………………………………

…………………………………

Visualisation   YES/NO

Creativity/Joy/Fun

…………………………………

…………………………………

Connection/Love

…………………………………

…………………………………

Priorities/Focus/Purpose

…………………………………

…………………………………

…………………………………

…………………………………

Date:………………………………..

Weight:…………………..

NUTRITION

Number of Meals…………

Protein	YES/NO
Fruit & vegetables	YES/NO
Healthy Fat	YES/NO
Fibre	YES/NO
Apple Cider Vinegar	YES/NO
Supplements	YES/NO

METABOLISM

Cold Exposure   YES/NO

Aerobic Exercise

✓   …………………

✓   …………………

Anaerobic Exercise

✓   …………………

✓   …………………

✓   …………………

✓   …………………

✓   …………………

✓   …………………

✓   …………………

Flexibility Exercise

✓   …………………

✓   …………………

TIMING

A Good Night's Sleep YES/NO

Breakfast...........................

Dinner Completed..............

Window...........................

Digital Curfew...................

Bedtime...........................

Date:.................................

Weight:......................

NUTRITION

Number of Meals............

Protein	YES/NO
Fruit & vegetables	YES/NO
Healthy Fat	YES/NO
Fibre	YES/NO
Apple Cider Vinegar	YES/NO
Supplements	YES/NO

MINDSET

Relaxation

....

....

Mindful Eating   YES/NO

Gratitude

....

....

....

Self-care & Kindness

....

....

Visualisation   YES/NO

Creativity/Joy/Fun

....

....

Connection/Love

....

....

Priorities/Focus/Purpose

....

....

....

....

METABOLISM

Cold Exposure   YES/NO

Aerobic Exercise

✓   ....

✓   ....

Anaerobic Exercise

✓   ....

✓   ....

✓   ....

✓   ....

✓   ....

✓   ....

✓   ....

Flexibility Exercise

✓   ....

✓   ....

TIMING

A Good Night's Sleep YES/NO

Breakfast...........................

Dinner Completed...............

Window...........................

Digital Curfew...................

Bedtime...........................

MINDSET

Relaxation
....
....

Mindful Eating   YES/NO

Gratitude
....
....
....

Self-care & Kindness
....
....

Visualisation   YES/NO

Creativity/Joy/Fun
....
....

Connection/Love
....
....

Priorities/Focus/Purpose
....
....
....
....

Date:................................

Weight:.....................

NUTRITION

Number of Meals............

Protein	YES/NO
Fruit & vegetables	YES/NO
Healthy Fat	YES/NO
Fibre	YES/NO
Apple Cider Vinegar	YES/NO
Supplements	YES/NO

METABOLISM

Cold Exposure   YES/NO

Aerobic Exercise
   ✓ ....
   ✓ ....

Anaerobic Exercise
   ✓ ....
   ✓ ....
   ✓ ....
   ✓ ....
   ✓ ....
   ✓ ....
   ✓ ....

Flexibility Exercise
   ✓ ....
   ✓ ....

WEEKLY REVIEW

Weight:

Review...........................

Weight:

Focus...............................

TIMING:

Review...............................
....
....
....
....

TIMING:

Focus...............................
....
....
....
....

MINDSET:

Review...............................
....
....
....
....
....
....

MINDSET:

Focus...............................
....
....
....
....
....
....

NUTRITION:

Review ....
....
....
....
....
....

NUTRITION:

Focus...............................
....
....
....
....
....

METABOLISM:

Review...............................
....
....
....
....

METABOLISM:

Focus...............................
....
....
....
....

"Every action needs to be prompted by a motive."

Leonardo Da Vinci

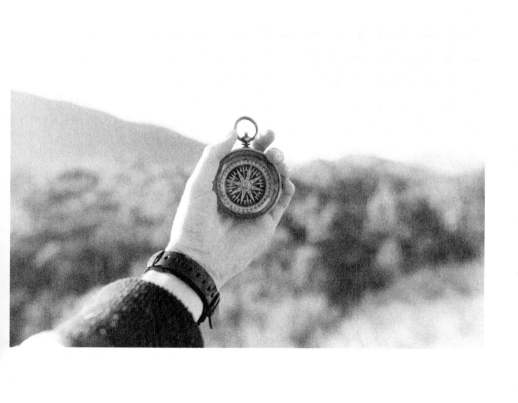

TIMING

A Good Night's Sleep YES/NO

Breakfast...........................

Dinner Completed...............

Window...........................

Digital Curfew....................

Bedtime...........................

MINDSET

Relaxation

....

....

Mindful Eating   YES/NO

Gratitude

....

....

....

Self-care & Kindness

....

....

Visualisation   YES/NO

Creativity/Joy/Fun

....

....

Connection/Love

....

....

Priorities/Focus/Purpose

....

....

....

....

Date:..............................

Weight:......................

NUTRITION

Number of Meals............

Protein	YES/NO
Fruit & vegetables	YES/NO
Healthy Fat	YES/NO
Fibre	YES/NO
Apple Cider Vinegar	YES/NO
Supplements	YES/NO

METABOLISM

Cold Exposure   YES/NO

Aerobic Exercise

   ✓   ....
   ✓   ....

Anaerobic Exercise

   ✓   ....
   ✓   ....
   ✓   ....
   ✓   ....
   ✓   ....
   ✓   ....
   ✓   ....

Flexibility Exercise

   ✓   ....
   ✓   ....

TIMING

A Good Night's Sleep YES/NO

Breakfast...........................

Dinner Completed...............

Window...........................

Digital Curfew..................

Bedtime...........................

MINDSET

Relaxation
....
....

Mindful Eating   YES/NO

Gratitude
....
....
....

Self-care & Kindness
....
....

Visualisation   YES/NO

Creativity/Joy/Fun
....
....

Connection/Love
....
....

Priorities/Focus/Purpose
....
....
....
....

Date:.............................

Weight:........................

NUTRITION

Number of Meals............

Protein	YES/NO
Fruit & vegetables	YES/NO
Healthy Fat	YES/NO
Fibre	YES/NO
Apple Cider Vinegar	YES/NO
Supplements	YES/NO

METABOLISM

Cold Exposure   YES/NO

Aerobic Exercise

   ✓   ....
   ✓   ....

Anaerobic Exercise

   ✓   ....
   ✓   ....
   ✓   ....
   ✓   ....
   ✓   ....
   ✓   ....
   ✓   ....

Flexibility Exercise

   ✓   ....
   ✓   ....

TIMING

A Good Night's Sleep YES/NO

Breakfast............................

Dinner Completed...............

Window............................

Digital Curfew...................

Bedtime............................

MINDSET

Relaxation

....

....

Mindful Eating   YES/NO

Gratitude

....

....

....

Self-care & Kindness

....

....

Visualisation   YES/NO

Creativity/Joy/Fun

....

....

Connection/Love

....

....

Priorities/Focus/Purpose

....

....

....

....

Date:.................................

Weight:.......................

NUTRITION

Number of Meals............

Protein	YES/NO
Fruit & vegetables	YES/NO
Healthy Fat	YES/NO
Fibre	YES/NO
Apple Cider Vinegar	YES/NO
Supplements	YES/NO

METABOLISM

Cold Exposure   YES/NO

Aerobic Exercise

✓ ....

✓ ....

Anaerobic Exercise

✓ ....

✓ ....

✓ ....

✓ ....

✓ ....

✓ ....

✓ ....

Flexibility Exercise

✓ ....

✓ ....

TIMING

A Good Night's Sleep YES/NO

Breakfast...........................

Dinner Completed..............

Window...........................

Digital Curfew...................

Bedtime...........................

MINDSET

Relaxation
....
....

Mindful Eating   YES/NO

Gratitude
....
....
....

Self-care & Kindness
....
....

Visualisation   YES/NO

Creativity/Joy/Fun
....
....

Connection/Love
....
....

Priorities/Focus/Purpose
....
....
....
....

Date:................................

Weight:......................

NUTRITION

Number of Meals............

Protein	YES/NO
Fruit & vegetables	YES/NO
Healthy Fat	YES/NO
Fibre	YES/NO
Apple Cider Vinegar	YES/NO
Supplements	YES/NO

METABOLISM

Cold Exposure   YES/NO

Aerobic Exercise
   ✓ ....
   ✓ ....

Anaerobic Exercise
   ✓ ....
   ✓ ....
   ✓ ....
   ✓ ....
   ✓ ....
   ✓ ....
   ✓ ....

Flexibility Exercise
   ✓ ....
   ✓ ....

TIMING

A Good Night's Sleep YES/NO

Breakfast.............................

Dinner Completed...............

Window..............................

Digital Curfew....................

Bedtime.............................

MINDSET

Relaxation
....
....

Mindful Eating   YES/NO

Gratitude
....
....
....

Self-care & Kindness
....
....

Visualisation   YES/NO

Creativity/Joy/Fun
....
....

Connection/Love
....
....

Priorities/Focus/Purpose
....
....
....
....

Date:................................

Weight:.......................

NUTRITION

Number of Meals.............

Protein	YES/NO
Fruit & vegetables	YES/NO
Healthy Fat	YES/NO
Fibre	YES/NO
Apple Cider Vinegar	YES/NO
Supplements	YES/NO

METABOLISM

Cold Exposure   YES/NO

Aerobic Exercise
✓ ....
✓ ....

Anaerobic Exercise
✓ ....
✓ ....
✓ ....
✓ ....
✓ ....
✓ ....
✓ ....

Flexibility Exercise
✓ ....
✓ ....

TIMING

A Good Night's Sleep YES/NO

Breakfast...........................

Dinner Completed...............

Window............................

Digital Curfew...................

Bedtime...........................

MINDSET

Relaxation
....
....

Mindful Eating   YES/NO

Gratitude
....
....
....

Self-care & Kindness
....
....

Visualisation   YES/NO

Creativity/Joy/Fun
....
....

Connection/Love
....
....

Priorities/Focus/Purpose
....
....
....
....

Date:................................

Weight:......................

NUTRITION

Number of Meals............

Protein	YES/NO
Fruit & vegetables	YES/NO
Healthy Fat	YES/NO
Fibre	YES/NO
Apple Cider Vinegar	YES/NO
Supplements	YES/NO

METABOLISM

Cold Exposure   YES/NO

Aerobic Exercise
   ✓ ....
   ✓ ....

Anaerobic Exercise
   ✓ ....
   ✓ ....
   ✓ ....
   ✓ ....
   ✓ ....
   ✓ ....
   ✓ ....

Flexibility Exercise
   ✓ ....
   ✓ ....

TIMING

A Good Night's Sleep YES/NO

Breakfast...........................

Dinner Completed...............

Window...........................

Digital Curfew...................

Bedtime...........................

MINDSET

Relaxation
....
....

Mindful Eating   YES/NO

Gratitude
....
....
....

Self-care & Kindness
....
....

Visualisation   YES/NO

Creativity/Joy/Fun
....
....

Connection/Love
....
....

Priorities/Focus/Purpose
....
....
....
....

Date:...............................

Weight:........................

NUTRITION

Number of Meals............

Protein   YES/NO

Fruit & vegetables   YES/NO

Healthy Fat   YES/NO

Fibre   YES/NO

Apple Cider Vinegar   YES/NO

Supplements   YES/NO

METABOLISM

Cold Exposure   YES/NO

Aerobic Exercise
 ✓ ....
 ✓ ....

Anaerobic Exercise
 ✓ ....
 ✓ ....
 ✓ ....
 ✓ ....
 ✓ ....
 ✓ ....
 ✓ ....

Flexibility Exercise
 ✓ ....
 ✓ ....

WEEKLY REVIEW

Weight:

Review.............................

Weight:

Focus..............................

TIMING:

Review.............................
....
....
....
....

TIMING:

Focus.................................
....
....
....
....

MINDSET:

Review.............................
....
....
....
....
....
....

MINDSET:

Focus.................................
....
....
....
....
....
....

NUTRITION:

Review ....
....
....
....
....
....

NUTRITION:

Focus.................................
....
....
....
....

METABOLISM:

Review.............................
....
....
....
....

METABOLISM:

Focus.................................
....
....
....
....

"It is not death that a man should fear, but he should fear never beginning to live."

Marcus Aurelius

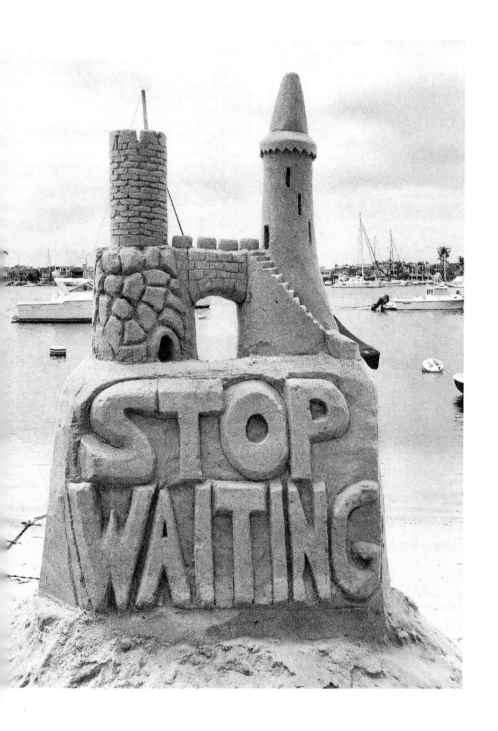

TIMING

A Good Night's Sleep YES/NO

Breakfast...........................

Dinner Completed...............

Window...........................

Digital Curfew...................

Bedtime...........................

MINDSET

Relaxation

....

....

Mindful Eating   YES/NO

Gratitude

....

....

....

Self-care & Kindness

....

....

Visualisation   YES/NO

Creativity/Joy/Fun

....

....

Connection/Love

....

....

Priorities/Focus/Purpose

....

....

....

....

Date:...............................

Weight:.......................

NUTRITION

Number of Meals............

Protein   YES/NO

Fruit & vegetables   YES/NO

Healthy Fat   YES/NO

Fibre   YES/NO

Apple Cider Vinegar   YES/NO

Supplements   YES/NO

METABOLISM

Cold Exposure   YES/NO

Aerobic Exercise

   ✓   ....
   ✓   ....

Anaerobic Exercise

   ✓   ....
   ✓   ....
   ✓   ....
   ✓   ....
   ✓   ....
   ✓   ....
   ✓   ....

Flexibility Exercise

   ✓   ....
   ✓   ....

TIMING

A Good Night's Sleep YES/NO

Breakfast...........................

Dinner Completed...............

Window...........................

Digital Curfew...................

Bedtime...........................

MINDSET

Relaxation

....

....

Mindful Eating   YES/NO

Gratitude

....

....

....

Self-care & Kindness

....

....

Visualisation   YES/NO

Creativity/Joy/Fun

....

....

Connection/Love

....

....

Priorities/Focus/Purpose

....

....

....

....

Date:..............................

Weight:.......................

NUTRITION

Number of Meals............

Protein	YES/NO
Fruit & vegetables	YES/NO
Healthy Fat	YES/NO
Fibre	YES/NO
Apple Cider Vinegar	YES/NO
Supplements	YES/NO

METABOLISM

Cold Exposure   YES/NO

Aerobic Exercise

✓   ....

✓   ....

Anaerobic Exercise

✓   ....

✓   ....

✓   ....

✓   ....

✓   ....

✓   ....

✓   ....

Flexibility Exercise

✓   ....

✓   ....

TIMING

A Good Night's Sleep YES/NO

Breakfast.............................

Dinner Completed...............

Window............................

Digital Curfew...................

Bedtime............................

MINDSET

Relaxation

....

....

Mindful Eating   YES/NO

Gratitude

....

....

....

Self-care & Kindness

....

....

Visualisation   YES/NO

Creativity/Joy/Fun

....

....

Connection/Love

....

....

Priorities/Focus/Purpose

....

....

....

....

Date:................................

Weight:.......................

NUTRITION

Number of Meals.............

Protein   YES/NO

Fruit & vegetables   YES/NO

Healthy Fat   YES/NO

Fibre   YES/NO

Apple Cider Vinegar   YES/NO

Supplements   YES/NO

METABOLISM

Cold Exposure   YES/NO

Aerobic Exercise

   ✓ ....

   ✓ ....

Anaerobic Exercise

   ✓ ....

   ✓ ....

   ✓ ....

   ✓ ....

   ✓ ....

   ✓ ....

   ✓ ....

Flexibility Exercise

   ✓ ....

   ✓ ....

TIMING

A Good Night's Sleep YES/NO

Breakfast...........................

Dinner Completed...............

Window............................

Digital Curfew...................

Bedtime............................

MINDSET

Relaxation
....
....

Mindful Eating   YES/NO

Gratitude
....
....
....

Self-care & Kindness
....
....

Visualisation   YES/NO

Creativity/Joy/Fun
....
....

Connection/Love
....
....

Priorities/Focus/Purpose
....
....
....
....

Date:...................................

Weight:........................

NUTRITION

Number of Meals............

Protein	YES/NO
Fruit & vegetables	YES/NO
Healthy Fat	YES/NO
Fibre	YES/NO
Apple Cider Vinegar	YES/NO
Supplements	YES/NO

METABOLISM

Cold Exposure   YES/NO

Aerobic Exercise
✓   ....
✓   ....

Anaerobic Exercise
✓   ....
✓   ....
✓   ....
✓   ....
✓   ....
✓   ....
✓   ....

Flexibility Exercise
✓   ....
✓   ....

TIMING

A Good Night's Sleep YES/NO

Breakfast...........................

Dinner Completed...............

Window...........................

Digital Curfew...................

Bedtime...........................

MINDSET

Relaxation
....
....

Mindful Eating   YES/NO

Gratitude
....
....
....

Self-care & Kindness
....
....

Visualisation   YES/NO

Creativity/Joy/Fun
....
....

Connection/Love
....
....

Priorities/Focus/Purpose
....
....
....
....

Date:...............................

Weight:.......................

NUTRITION

Number of Meals............

Protein	YES/NO
Fruit & vegetables	YES/NO
Healthy Fat	YES/NO
Fibre	YES/NO
Apple Cider Vinegar	YES/NO
Supplements	YES/NO

METABOLISM

Cold Exposure   YES/NO

Aerobic Exercise
  ✓ ....
  ✓ ....

Anaerobic Exercise
  ✓ ....
  ✓ ....
  ✓ ....
  ✓ ....
  ✓ ....
  ✓ ....
  ✓ ....

Flexibility Exercise
  ✓ ....
  ✓ ....

TIMING

A Good Night's Sleep YES/NO

Breakfast...........................

Dinner Completed...............

Window...........................

Digital Curfew...................

Bedtime...........................

MINDSET

Relaxation

....
....

Mindful Eating   YES/NO

Gratitude

....
....
....

Self-care & Kindness

....
....

Visualisation   YES/NO

Creativity/Joy/Fun

....
....

Connection/Love

....
....

Priorities/Focus/Purpose

....
....
....
....

Date:..............................

Weight:.......................

NUTRITION

Number of Meals............

Protein	YES/NO
Fruit & vegetables	YES/NO
Healthy Fat	YES/NO
Fibre	YES/NO
Apple Cider Vinegar	YES/NO
Supplements	YES/NO

METABOLISM

Cold Exposure   YES/NO

Aerobic Exercise

✓   ....
✓   ....

Anaerobic Exercise

✓   ....
✓   ....
✓   ....
✓   ....
✓   ....
✓   ....
✓   ....

Flexibility Exercise

✓   ....
✓   ....

TIMING

A Good Night's Sleep YES/NO

Breakfast...........................

Dinner Completed...............

Window............................

Digital Curfew....................

Bedtime............................

MINDSET

Relaxation

....

....

Mindful Eating   YES/NO

Gratitude

....

....

....

Self-care & Kindness

....

....

Visualisation   YES/NO

Creativity/Joy/Fun

....

....

Connection/Love

....

....

Priorities/Focus/Purpose

....

....

....

....

Date:............................

Weight:........................

NUTRITION

Number of Meals.............

Protein	YES/NO
Fruit & vegetables	YES/NO
Healthy Fat	YES/NO
Fibre	YES/NO
Apple Cider Vinegar	YES/NO
Supplements	YES/NO

METABOLISM

Cold Exposure   YES/NO

Aerobic Exercise

   ✓   ....

   ✓   ....

Anaerobic Exercise

   ✓   ....

   ✓   ....

   ✓   ....

   ✓   ....

   ✓   ....

   ✓   ....

   ✓   ....

Flexibility Exercise

   ✓   ....

   ✓   ....

WEEKLY REVIEW

Weight:	**Weight:**
Review............................	Focus............................

TIMING:	**TIMING:**
Review...........................	Focus............................
....	....
....	....
....	....
....	....

MINDSET:	**MINDSET:**
Review...........................	Focus............................
....	....
....	....
....	....
....	....
....	....
....	....

NUTRITION:	**NUTRITION:**
Review...........................	Focus............................
....	....
....	....
....	....
....	....
....	....

METABOLISM:	**METABOLISM:**
Review...........................	Focus............................
....	....
....	....
....	....
....	....

"The promises of this world are, for the most part, vain phantoms; and to confide in one's self, and become something of worth and value is the best and safest course."

Michelangelo

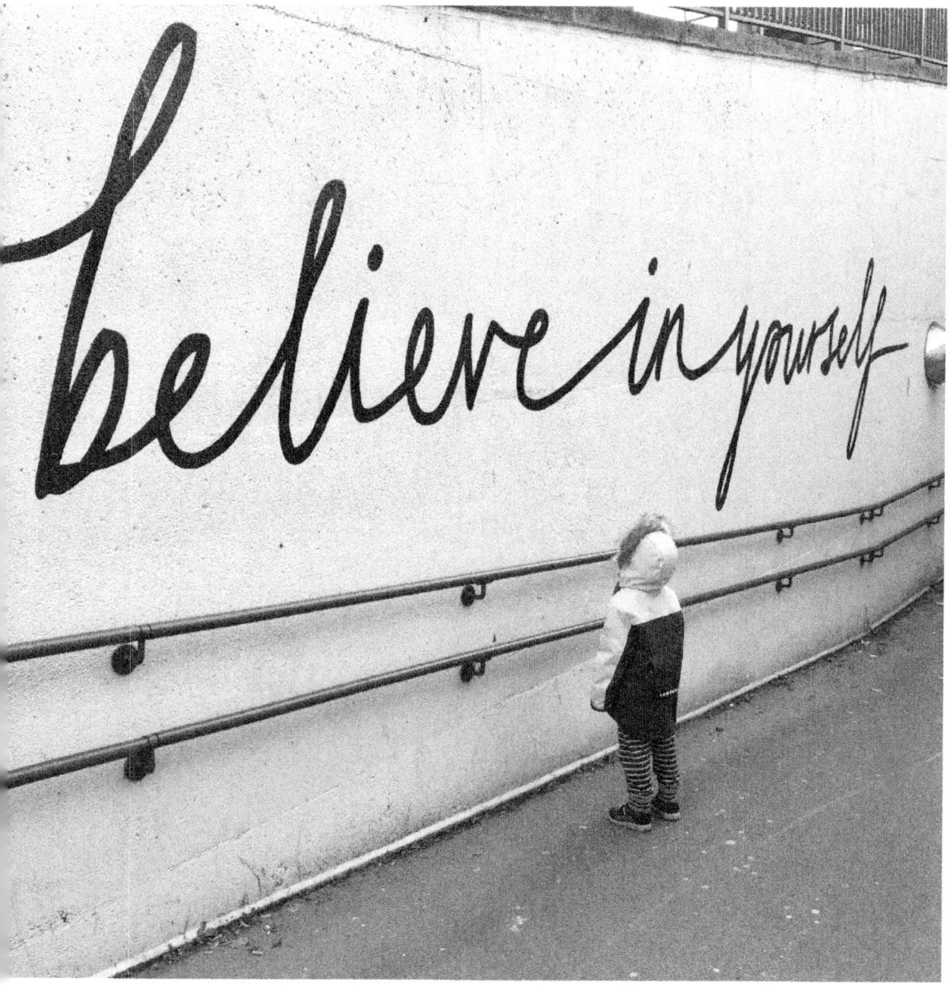
believe in yourself

TIMING

A Good Night's Sleep YES/NO

Breakfast...........................

Dinner Completed...............

Window...........................

Digital Curfew...................

Bedtime...........................

MINDSET

Relaxation
....
....

Mindful Eating   YES/NO

Gratitude
....
....
....

Self-care & Kindness
....
....

Visualisation   YES/NO

Creativity/Joy/Fun
....
....

Connection/Love
....
....

Priorities/Focus/Purpose
....
....
....
....

Date:.................................

Weight:.......................

NUTRITION

Number of Meals............

Protein	YES/NO
Fruit & vegetables	YES/NO
Healthy Fat	YES/NO
Fibre	YES/NO
Apple Cider Vinegar	YES/NO
Supplements	YES/NO

METABOLISM

Cold Exposure   YES/NO

Aerobic Exercise
   ✓ ....
   ✓ ....

Anaerobic Exercise
   ✓ ....
   ✓ ....
   ✓ ....
   ✓ ....
   ✓ ....
   ✓ ....
   ✓ ....

Flexibility Exercise
   ✓ ....
   ✓ ....

TIMING

A Good Night's Sleep YES/NO

Breakfast............................

Dinner Completed...............

Window...........................

Digital Curfew....................

Bedtime...........................

MINDSET

Relaxation

....

....

Mindful Eating   YES/NO

Gratitude

....

....

....

Self-care & Kindness

....

....

Visualisation   YES/NO

Creativity/Joy/Fun

....

....

Connection/Love

....

....

Priorities/Focus/Purpose

....

....

....

....

Date:...............................

Weight:.......................

NUTRITION

Number of Meals............	
Protein	YES/NO
Fruit & vegetables	YES/NO
Healthy Fat	YES/NO
Fibre	YES/NO
Apple Cider Vinegar	YES/NO
Supplements	YES/NO

METABOLISM

Cold Exposure   YES/NO

Aerobic Exercise

   ✓   ....
   ✓   ....

Anaerobic Exercise

   ✓   ....
   ✓   ....
   ✓   ....
   ✓   ....
   ✓   ....
   ✓   ....
   ✓   ....

Flexibility Exercise

   ✓   ....
   ✓   ....

TIMING

A Good Night's Sleep YES/NO

Breakfast...........................

Dinner Completed................

Window............................

Digital Curfew....................

Bedtime...........................

MINDSET

Relaxation
....
....

Mindful Eating   YES/NO

Gratitude
....
....
....

Self-care & Kindness
....
....

Visualisation   YES/NO

Creativity/Joy/Fun
....
....

Connection/Love
....
....

Priorities/Focus/Purpose
....
....
....
....

Date:............................…..

Weight:........................…..

NUTRITION

Number of Meals.............

Protein	YES/NO
Fruit & vegetables	YES/NO
Healthy Fat	YES/NO
Fibre	YES/NO
Apple Cider Vinegar	YES/NO
Supplements	YES/NO

METABOLISM

Cold Exposure   YES/NO

Aerobic Exercise
   ✓   ....
   ✓   ....

Anaerobic Exercise
   ✓   ....
   ✓   ....
   ✓   ....
   ✓   ....
   ✓   ....
   ✓   ....
   ✓   ....

Flexibility Exercise
   ✓   ....
   ✓   ....

TIMING

A Good Night's Sleep YES/NO

Breakfast............................

Dinner Completed...............

Window...........................

Digital Curfew...................

Bedtime...........................

MINDSET

Relaxation
....
....

Mindful Eating   YES/NO

Gratitude
....
....
....

Self-care & Kindness
....
....

Visualisation   YES/NO

Creativity/Joy/Fun
....
....

Connection/Love
....
....

Priorities/Focus/Purpose
....
....
....
....

Date:................................

Weight:......................

NUTRITION

Number of Meals............

Protein	YES/NO
Fruit & vegetables	YES/NO
Healthy Fat	YES/NO
Fibre	YES/NO
Apple Cider Vinegar	YES/NO
Supplements	YES/NO

METABOLISM

Cold Exposure   YES/NO

Aerobic Exercise
  ✓   ....
  ✓   ....

Anaerobic Exercise
  ✓   ....
  ✓   ....
  ✓   ....
  ✓   ....
  ✓   ....
  ✓   ....
  ✓   ....

Flexibility Exercise
  ✓   ....
  ✓   ....

TIMING

A Good Night's Sleep YES/NO

Breakfast............................

Dinner Completed...............

Window............................

Digital Curfew...................

Bedtime............................

MINDSET

Relaxation
....
....

Mindful Eating   YES/NO

Gratitude
....
....
....

Self-care & Kindness
....
....

Visualisation   YES/NO

Creativity/Joy/Fun
....
....

Connection/Love
....
....

Priorities/Focus/Purpose
....
....
....
....

Date:................................

Weight:.......................

NUTRITION

Number of Meals............

Protein   YES/NO

Fruit & vegetables   YES/NO

Healthy Fat   YES/NO

Fibre   YES/NO

Apple Cider Vinegar   YES/NO

Supplements   YES/NO

METABOLISM

Cold Exposure   YES/NO

Aerobic Exercise

✓   ....
✓   ....

Anaerobic Exercise

✓   ....
✓   ....
✓   ....
✓   ....
✓   ....
✓   ....
✓   ....

Flexibility Exercise

✓   ....
✓   ....

TIMING

A Good Night's Sleep YES/NO

Breakfast............................

Dinner Completed...............

Window...........................

Digital Curfew...................

Bedtime...........................

MINDSET

Relaxation
....
....

Mindful Eating   YES/NO

Gratitude
....
....
....

Self-care & Kindness
....
....

Visualisation   YES/NO

Creativity/Joy/Fun
....
....

Connection/Love
....
....

Priorities/Focus/Purpose
....
....
....
....

Date:...............................

Weight:.......................

NUTRITION

Number of Meals............

Protein	YES/NO
Fruit & vegetables	YES/NO
Healthy Fat	YES/NO
Fibre	YES/NO
Apple Cider Vinegar	YES/NO
Supplements	YES/NO

METABOLISM

Cold Exposure   YES/NO

Aerobic Exercise
✓ ....
✓ ....

Anaerobic Exercise
✓ ....
✓ ....
✓ ....
✓ ....
✓ ....
✓ ....
✓ ....

Flexibility Exercise
✓ ....
✓ ....

TIMING

A Good Night's Sleep YES/NO

Breakfast...........................

Dinner Completed...............

Window...........................

Digital Curfew...................

Bedtime...........................

MINDSET

Relaxation

....

....

Mindful Eating   YES/NO

Gratitude

....

....

....

Self-care & Kindness

....

....

Visualisation   YES/NO

Creativity/Joy/Fun

....

....

Connection/Love

....

....

Priorities/Focus/Purpose

....

....

....

....

Date:................................

Weight:......................

NUTRITION

Number of Meals............

Protein   YES/NO

Fruit & vegetables   YES/NO

Healthy Fat   YES/NO

Fibre   YES/NO

Apple Cider Vinegar   YES/NO

Supplements   YES/NO

METABOLISM

Cold Exposure   YES/NO

Aerobic Exercise

✓ ....

✓ ....

Anaerobic Exercise

✓ ....

✓ ....

✓ ....

✓ ....

✓ ....

✓ ....

✓ ....

Flexibility Exercise

✓ ....

✓ ....

WEEKLY REVIEW

Weight:

Review...............................

Weight:

Focus...............................

TIMING:

Review...............................
....
....
....
....

TIMING:

Focus...............................
....
....
....
....

MINDSET:

Review...............................
....
....
....
....
....
....

MINDSET:

Focus...............................
....
....
....
....
....
....

NUTRITION:

Review ....
....
....
....
....
....

NUTRITION:

Focus...............................
....
....
....
....

METABOLISM:

Review...............................
....
....
....
....

METABOLISM:

Focus...............................
....
....
....

"People in their handlings of affairs often fail when they are about to succeed. If one remains as careful at the end as he was at the beginning, there will be no failure."

Lao Tzu

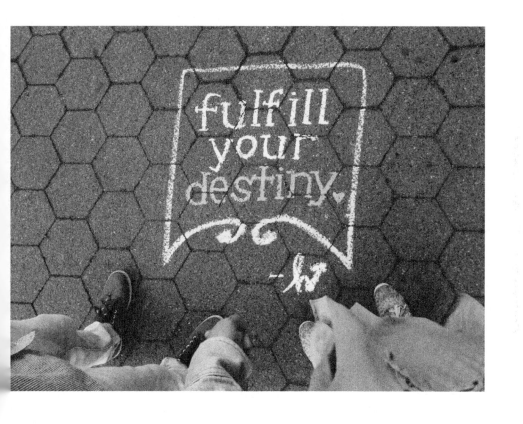

TIMING

A Good Night's Sleep YES/NO

Breakfast...........................

Dinner Completed...............

Window...........................

Digital Curfew...................

Bedtime...........................

MINDSET

Relaxation

....

....

Mindful Eating   YES/NO

Gratitude

....

....

....

Self-care & Kindness

....

....

Visualisation   YES/NO

Creativity/Joy/Fun

....

....

Connection/Love

....

....

Priorities/Focus/Purpose

....

....

....

....

Date:................................

Weight:......................

NUTRITION

Number of Meals............

Protein   YES/NO

Fruit & vegetables   YES/NO

Healthy Fat   YES/NO

Fibre   YES/NO

Apple Cider Vinegar   YES/NO

Supplements   YES/NO

METABOLISM

Cold Exposure   YES/NO

Aerobic Exercise

✓ ....

✓ ....

Anaerobic Exercise

✓ ....

✓ ....

✓ ....

✓ ....

✓ ....

✓ ....

✓ ....

Flexibility Exercise

✓ ....

✓ ....

TIMING

A Good Night's Sleep YES/NO

Breakfast...........................

Dinner Completed...............

Window...........................

Digital Curfew...................

Bedtime...........................

MINDSET

Relaxation

....

....

Mindful Eating   YES/NO

Gratitude

....

....

....

Self-care & Kindness

....

....

Visualisation   YES/NO

Creativity/Joy/Fun

....

....

Connection/Love

....

....

Priorities/Focus/Purpose

....

....

....

....

Date:...............................

Weight:.......................

NUTRITION

Number of Meals............

Protein	YES/NO
Fruit & vegetables	YES/NO
Healthy Fat	YES/NO
Fibre	YES/NO
Apple Cider Vinegar	YES/NO
Supplements	YES/NO

METABOLISM

Cold Exposure   YES/NO

Aerobic Exercise

✓   ....

✓   ....

Anaerobic Exercise

✓   ....

✓   ....

✓   ....

✓   ....

✓   ....

✓   ....

✓   ....

Flexibility Exercise

✓   ....

✓   ....

TIMING

A Good Night's Sleep YES/NO

Breakfast...........................

Dinner Completed...............

Window........................

Digital Curfew..................

Bedtime..........................

MINDSET

Relaxation
....
....

Mindful Eating   YES/NO

Gratitude
....
....
....

Self-care & Kindness
....
....

Visualisation   YES/NO

Creativity/Joy/Fun
....
....

Connection/Love
....
....

Priorities/Focus/Purpose
....
....
....
....

Date:.................................

Weight:......................

NUTRITION

Number of Meals............

Protein	YES/NO
Fruit & vegetables	YES/NO
Healthy Fat	YES/NO
Fibre	YES/NO
Apple Cider Vinegar	YES/NO
Supplements	YES/NO

METABOLISM

Cold Exposure   YES/NO

Aerobic Exercise
  ✓ ....
  ✓ ....

Anaerobic Exercise
  ✓ ....
  ✓ ....
  ✓ ....
  ✓ ....
  ✓ ....
  ✓ ....
  ✓ ....

Flexibility Exercise
  ✓ ....
  ✓ ....

TIMING

A Good Night's Sleep YES/NO

Breakfast..........................

Dinner Completed...............

Window...........................

Digital Curfew...................

Bedtime...........................

MINDSET

Relaxation

....

....

Mindful Eating   YES/NO

Gratitude

....

....

....

Self-care & Kindness

....

....

Visualisation   YES/NO

Creativity/Joy/Fun

....

....

Connection/Love

....

....

Priorities/Focus/Purpose

....

....

....

....

Date:.............................

Weight:........................

NUTRITION

Number of Meals............

Protein   YES/NO

Fruit & vegetables   YES/NO

Healthy Fat   YES/NO

Fibre   YES/NO

Apple Cider Vinegar   YES/NO

Supplements   YES/NO

METABOLISM

Cold Exposure   YES/NO

Aerobic Exercise

✓   ....

✓   ....

Anaerobic Exercise

✓   ....

✓   ....

✓   ....

✓   ....

✓   ....

✓   ....

✓   ....

Flexibility Exercise

✓   ....

✓   ....

TIMING

A Good Night's Sleep YES/NO

Breakfast...........................

Dinner Completed...............

Window............................

Digital Curfew...................

Bedtime...........................

MINDSET

Relaxation

....
....

Mindful Eating   YES/NO

Gratitude

....
....
....

Self-care & Kindness

....
....

Visualisation   YES/NO

Creativity/Joy/Fun

....
....

Connection/Love

....
....

Priorities/Focus/Purpose

....
....
....
....

Date:...............................

Weight:........................

NUTRITION

Number of Meals............

Protein   YES/NO

Fruit & vegetables   YES/NO

Healthy Fat   YES/NO

Fibre   YES/NO

Apple Cider Vinegar   YES/NO

Supplements   YES/NO

METABOLISM

Cold Exposure   YES/NO

Aerobic Exercise

   ✓   ....
   ✓   ....

Anaerobic Exercise

   ✓   ....
   ✓   ....
   ✓   ....
   ✓   ....
   ✓   ....
   ✓   ....
   ✓   ....

Flexibility Exercise

   ✓   ....
   ✓   ....

TIMING

A Good Night's Sleep YES/NO

Breakfast..........................

Dinner Completed...............

Window.........................

Digital Curfew..................

Bedtime..........................

MINDSET

Relaxation
....
....

Mindful Eating   YES/NO

Gratitude
....
....
....

Self-care & Kindness
....
....

Visualisation   YES/NO

Creativity/Joy/Fun
....
....

Connection/Love
....
....

Priorities/Focus/Purpose
....
....
....
....

Date:.................................

Weight:.....................

NUTRITION

Number of Meals............

Protein	YES/NO
Fruit & vegetables	YES/NO
Healthy Fat	YES/NO
Fibre	YES/NO
Apple Cider Vinegar	YES/NO
Supplements	YES/NO

METABOLISM

Cold Exposure   YES/NO

Aerobic Exercise
✓ ....
✓ ....

Anaerobic Exercise
✓ ....
✓ ....
✓ ....
✓ ....
✓ ....
✓ ....
✓ ....

Flexibility Exercise
✓ ....
✓ ....

TIMING

A Good Night's Sleep YES/NO

Breakfast.............................

Dinner Completed................

Window.............................

Digital Curfew....................

Bedtime.............................

MINDSET

Relaxation
....
....

Mindful Eating YES/NO

Gratitude
....
....
....

Self-care & Kindness
....
....

Visualisation YES/NO

Creativity/Joy/Fun
....
....

Connection/Love
....
....

Priorities/Focus/Purpose
....
....
....
....

Date:................................

Weight:.......................

NUTRITION

Number of Meals.............

Protein	YES/NO
Fruit & vegetables	YES/NO
Healthy Fat	YES/NO
Fibre	YES/NO
Apple Cider Vinegar	YES/NO
Supplements	YES/NO

METABOLISM

Cold Exposure YES/NO

Aerobic Exercise
✓ ....
✓ ....

Anaerobic Exercise
✓ ....
✓ ....
✓ ....
✓ ....
✓ ....
✓ ....
✓ ....

Flexibility Exercise
✓ ....
✓ ....

WEEKLY REVIEW

Weight:

Review.............................

Weight:

Focus................................

TIMING:

Review.............................
....
....
....
....

TIMING:

Focus...............................
....
....
....

MINDSET:

Review.............................
....
....
....
....
....
....

MINDSET:

Focus................................
....
....
....
....
....
....

NUTRITION:

Review ....
....
....
....
....
....

NUTRITION:

Focus................................
....
....
....
....

METABOLISM:

Review.............................
....
....
....
....

METABOLISM:

Focus................................
....
....
....
....

"Today you are you! That is truer than true! There is no one alive who is you-er than you!"

Dr. Seuss

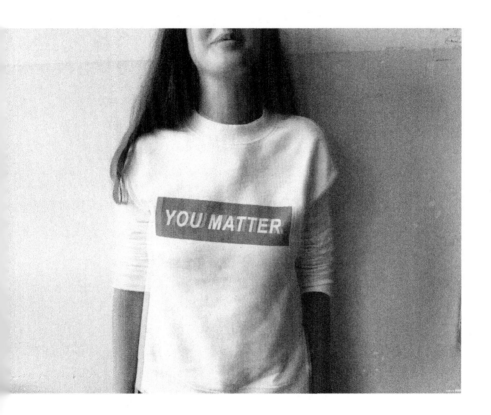

TIMING

A Good Night's Sleep YES/NO

Breakfast..........................

Dinner Completed...............

Window...........................

Digital Curfew...................

Bedtime...........................

MINDSET

Relaxation

....

....

Mindful Eating   YES/NO

Gratitude

....

....

....

Self-care & Kindness

....

....

Visualisation   YES/NO

Creativity/Joy/Fun

....

....

Connection/Love

....

....

Priorities/Focus/Purpose

....

....

....

....

Date:.................................

Weight:.......................

NUTRITION

Number of Meals............

Protein   YES/NO

Fruit & vegetables   YES/NO

Healthy Fat   YES/NO

Fibre   YES/NO

Apple Cider Vinegar   YES/NO

Supplements   YES/NO

METABOLISM

Cold Exposure   YES/NO

Aerobic Exercise

    ✓   ....
    ✓   ....

Anaerobic Exercise

    ✓   ....
    ✓   ....
    ✓   ....
    ✓   ....
    ✓   ....
    ✓   ....
    ✓   ....

Flexibility Exercise

    ✓   ....
    ✓   ....

TIMING

A Good Night's Sleep YES/NO

Breakfast...........................

Dinner Completed...............

Window...........................

Digital Curfew...................

Bedtime...........................

MINDSET

Relaxation

....

....

Mindful Eating   YES/NO

Gratitude

....

....

....

Self-care & Kindness

....

....

Visualisation   YES/NO

Creativity/Joy/Fun

....

....

Connection/Love

....

....

Priorities/Focus/Purpose

....

....

....

....

Date:...............................

Weight:......................

NUTRITION

Number of Meals............

Protein	YES/NO
Fruit & vegetables	YES/NO
Healthy Fat	YES/NO
Fibre	YES/NO
Apple Cider Vinegar	YES/NO
Supplements	YES/NO

METABOLISM

Cold Exposure   YES/NO

Aerobic Exercise

✓   ....
✓   ....

Anaerobic Exercise

✓   ....
✓   ....
✓   ....
✓   ....
✓   ....
✓   ....
✓   ....

Flexibility Exercise

✓   ....
✓   ....

TIMING

A Good Night's Sleep YES/NO

Breakfast...........................

Dinner Completed...............

Window...........................

Digital Curfew...................

Bedtime............................

MINDSET

Relaxation

....
....

Mindful Eating   YES/NO

Gratitude

....
....
....

Self-care & Kindness

....
....

Visualisation   YES/NO

Creativity/Joy/Fun

....
....

Connection/Love

....
....

Priorities/Focus/Purpose

....
....
....
....

Date:................................

Weight:.......................

NUTRITION

Number of Meals............

Protein   YES/NO

Fruit & vegetables   YES/NO

Healthy Fat   YES/NO

Fibre   YES/NO

Apple Cider Vinegar   YES/NO

Supplements   YES/NO

METABOLISM

Cold Exposure   YES/NO

Aerobic Exercise

✓   ....
✓   ....

Anaerobic Exercise

✓   ....
✓   ....
✓   ....
✓   ....
✓   ....
✓   ....
✓   ....

Flexibility Exercise

✓   ....
✓   ....

TIMING

A Good Night's Sleep YES/NO

Breakfast...........................

Dinner Completed...............

Window...........................

Digital Curfew..................

Bedtime...........................

MINDSET

Relaxation
....
....

Mindful Eating   YES/NO

Gratitude
....
....
....

Self-care & Kindness
....
....

Visualisation   YES/NO

Creativity/Joy/Fun
....
....

Connection/Love
....
....

Priorities/Focus/Purpose
....
....
....
....

Date:................................

Weight:.......................

NUTRITION

Number of Meals............

Protein	YES/NO
Fruit & vegetables	YES/NO
Healthy Fat	YES/NO
Fibre	YES/NO
Apple Cider Vinegar	YES/NO
Supplements	YES/NO

METABOLISM

Cold Exposure   YES/NO

Aerobic Exercise

   ✓ ....
   ✓ ....

Anaerobic Exercise

   ✓ ....
   ✓ ....
   ✓ ....
   ✓ ....
   ✓ ....
   ✓ ....
   ✓ ....

Flexibility Exercise

   ✓ ....
   ✓ ....

TIMING

A Good Night's Sleep YES/NO

Breakfast...........................

Dinner Completed...............

Window...........................

Digital Curfew...................

Bedtime...........................

Date:.................................

Weight:.......................

NUTRITION

Number of Meals............

Protein	YES/NO
Fruit & vegetables	YES/NO
Healthy Fat	YES/NO
Fibre	YES/NO
Apple Cider Vinegar	YES/NO
Supplements	YES/NO

MINDSET

Relaxation
....
....

Mindful Eating   YES/NO

Gratitude
....
....
....

Self-care & Kindness
....
....

Visualisation   YES/NO

Creativity/Joy/Fun
....
....

Connection/Love
....
....

Priorities/Focus/Purpose
....
....
....
....

METABOLISM

Cold Exposure   YES/NO

Aerobic Exercise

✓   ....
✓   ....

Anaerobic Exercise

✓   ....
✓   ....
✓   ....
✓   ....
✓   ....
✓   ....
✓   ....

Flexibility Exercise

✓   ....
✓   ....

TIMING

A Good Night's Sleep YES/NO

Breakfast...........................

Dinner Completed...............

Window...........................

Digital Curfew...................

Bedtime...........................

MINDSET

Relaxation

....
....

Mindful Eating   YES/NO

Gratitude

....
....
....

Self-care & Kindness

....
....

Visualisation   YES/NO

Creativity/Joy/Fun

....
....

Connection/Love

....
....

Priorities/Focus/Purpose

....
....
....
....

Date:................................

Weight:........................

NUTRITION

Number of Meals............

Protein	YES/NO
Fruit & vegetables	YES/NO
Healthy Fat	YES/NO
Fibre	YES/NO
Apple Cider Vinegar	YES/NO
Supplements	YES/NO

METABOLISM

Cold Exposure   YES/NO

Aerobic Exercise

✓   ....
✓   ....

Anaerobic Exercise

✓   ....
✓   ....
✓   ....
✓   ....
✓   ....
✓   ....
✓   ....

Flexibility Exercise

✓   ....
✓   ....

TIMING

A Good Night's Sleep YES/NO

Breakfast...........................

Dinner Completed...............

Window............................

Digital Curfew....................

Bedtime............................

MINDSET

Relaxation
....
....

Mindful Eating   YES/NO

Gratitude
....
....
....

Self-care & Kindness
....
....

Visualisation   YES/NO

Creativity/Joy/Fun
....
....

Connection/Love
....
....

Priorities/Focus/Purpose
....
....
....
....

Date:...............................

Weight:.......................

NUTRITION

Number of Meals............

Protein   YES/NO

Fruit & vegetables   YES/NO

Healthy Fat   YES/NO

Fibre   YES/NO

Apple Cider Vinegar   YES/NO

Supplements   YES/NO

METABOLISM

Cold Exposure   YES/NO

Aerobic Exercise
   ✓   ....
   ✓   ....

Anaerobic Exercise
   ✓   ....
   ✓   ....
   ✓   ....
   ✓   ....
   ✓   ....
   ✓   ....
   ✓   ....

Flexibility Exercise
   ✓   ....
   ✓   ....

WEEKLY REVIEW

| Weight: | Weight: |
| Review............................. | Focus............................... |

TIMING:	TIMING:
Review............................	Focus.............................
....	....
....	....
....	....
....	....

MINDSET:	MINDSET:
Review............................	Focus..............................
....	....
....	....
....	....
....	....
....	....
....	....

NUTRITION:	NUTRITION:
Review	Focus.............................
....	....
....	....
....	....
....	....
....	....

METABOLISM:	METABOLISM:
Review............................	Focus.............................
....	....
....	....
....	....
....	....

FINAL REVIEW AND NEW FOCUS

_____

_____

_____

_____

_____

_____

_____

_____

_____

_____

_____

_____

_____

_____

_____

_____

_____

_____

"Still round the corner there
may wait,
A new road or a secret gate."

J. R. R. Tolkien

Printed in Great Britain
by Amazon

78304480R00153